GETTING IT STRAIGHT

The Norris Technique of Body Alignment

PATRICIA NORRIS

Getting it Straight

The Norris Technique of Body Alignment

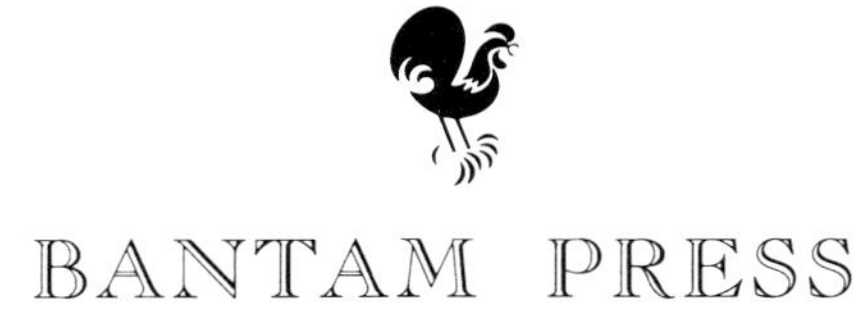

BANTAM PRESS
NEW YORK · LONDON · TORONTO · SYDNEY · AUCKLAND

TRANSWORLD PUBLISHERS LTD
61–63 Uxbridge Road, London W5 5SA

TRANSWORLD PUBLISHERS (AUSTRALIA) PTY LTD
26 Harley Crescent, Condell Park, NSW 2200

TRANSWORLD PUBLISHERS (NZ) LTD
Cnr. Moselle & Waipareira Aves,
Henderson, Auckland

Published 1986 by Bantam Press,
a division of Transworld Publishers Ltd

Photographs by Darryl Williams

British Library Cataloguing in Publication Data

Norris, Patricia
Getting it straight: the Norris technique of body alignment.
1. Exercise 2. Physical fitness
I. Title
613.7′1 RA781

ISBN 0-593-01005-1
ISBN 0-593-01009-4 Pbk

Printed and bound in West Germany by
Mohndruck Graphische Betriebe GmbH, Gütersloh

To Roy, with love and appreciation
for his continual help.

GETTING IT STRAIGHT

The Norris Technique of Body Alignment

CONTENTS

INTRODUCTION

To most people, that fantastic machine we call the body is a big mystery. Despite the boom in the body-building business and a national addiction to sport and city marathons, few people understand how their body works or how to use it well.

The annual crop of 'how to pull yourself together' books offers a hundred different ways to run, swim, dance or jog yourself into condition, but doesn't show you how to improve your body position so that you move correctly. There may be references to the need for 'good posture' but the means of achieving this are never made completely clear.

Parents and teachers also recognize the need for 'good posture' but, well intentioned as they are, they may do more harm than good. They tell children not to slump and to sit up straight, but they don't tell them *how* to do it. Attempts to straighten often make things worse.

This book *does* tell you how. It tells you not only how to sit and stand straight, but also how to free your body from the pressures of a cramped posture so that every movement you make keeps you flexible and free from strain.

I prefer not to use the word *posture*, because it does not describe my work accurately. Posture implies posing, and that is not what I teach. My work consists of re-educating the body into a correct line-up of the parts, hence the name 'body alignment'.

In studying my technique, the Norris Alignment, you will learn how the body hinges together as a whole and how the misuse of one joint or group of muscles can cause pressure and pain elsewhere. You will also learn how the alignment of your body is governed by the position of your feet.

Correct positioning of the feet is vital

Working out the relationship of the feet to the rest of the body was the most important breakthrough in my search for a practical way to change how we use our bodies. My method is unique because I show you how to position your feet so that they do not sabotage the rest of your alignment; and because I teach you not only how to *stand* straight but also how to align your body correctly from the feet upwards during *movement*.

This is why I have been able to help so many sportsmen and sportswomen – golfers, skiers, swimmers, cyclists, tennis players – to improve their performance simply by changing the way they use their bodies.

People often tell me how much they enjoy fast, vigorous exercise. I believe them. The pleasure principle is marvellous. I heartily approve of it myself. But if your body alignment is wrong to start with it is not a good idea to build muscle on to it.

Bad habits like hunched shoulders, a hollow back or splayed feet will not only inhibit every movement you make but also put pressure on your joints and muscles, making them vulnerable to injury. Strenuous activities like sport or rigorous keep-fit routines increase the risk.

Re-align your body before you exercise

Re-aligning your body correctly beforehand will double the effectiveness of any exercise you take and enable you to build muscle to reinforce your good body position. It will also increase the pleasure of every movement you make for the rest of your life.

From my own early training in ballet I know that dancers have to sacrifice their bodies to their art, just as professional sportsmen and sportswomen often have to sacrifice their bodies to be competitive. For them I recommend the Norris Alignment exercises to counteract the adverse effects of pushing themselves to the limit.

For those of you who lead less dedicated lives, this book will put you in touch with your body and show you how to improve the way you use it. If the very thought of exercising until your muscles burn makes you reach for another cream cake, stay with me. This book is for you too.

The Norris Alignment technique is not just for the keep-fit fraternity. It is for everybody. Whatever your condition – in training or out of it, slim or overweight, young or old – it will make you look better and feel better, physically and psychologically.

People often ask me if it is too late to do anything to improve their bodies. I tell them about one of my older students, a charming, retired brigadier in his seventies. Using my techniques and exercises has not changed his silver locks into gold – magic is not what this work is about – but he *is* flexible in both body and mind and the most vigorous seventy-plus going on sixty you could meet.

You will look more attractive instantly

For both men and women the immediate effects of re-alignment are dramatic. Standing in the correct basic stance with the body stretched into an upward, thrusting, vertical position instantly reshapes the figure.

If you have a double chin or 'dowager's hump', it can be corrected. Your waistline is reduced and your stomach flattened. Your hip-line will appear slimmer. You will look taller. Best of all, you will look more attractive and more *alive*.

Here is a short list of the nice things that will happen to you when you know how to stand straight and square on your own two feet (I'll explain that later). Your new alignment will

— Tighten your face muscles
— Remove any double chin
— Lengthen the neck
— Correct 'dowager's hump'
— Slim your waist
— Flatten your stomach
— Firm outer thighs
— Tuck in your buttocks
— Slim your hip-line

— Increase your height
— Rejuvenate your figure

At the end of my classes people come to me and say how marvellous they feel. They look it too. They arrive with stooped shoulders, chins down and rears out. They leave moving with ease and fluency and with their bodies straight.

If you have recently lost weight, alignment exercises will help lift sagging muscles and re-contour your body. As we all know, losing weight is only half the battle. You still have to keep the weight off *and* transform that old fat shape into a thin one.

If you are overweight and you/your husband/wife/lover like you that way, re-alignment will help to redistribute your weight so that it is better balanced. In any case, stretching your body upwards will make you look much slimmer. If you do the 'bounces' I recommend every morning, they will not only gently exercise your heart and lungs but also help to stabilize your weight.

Apart from these simple bounces, there are no fast, repetitive exercise routines to do. You do not have to use any apparatus. You do not have to rely on being manipulated by someone else. Even if you do no other form of exercise or sport, what you learn to do in this book can strengthen your muscles and keep your body flexible.

What incorrect body alignment does to you

We all tend to bring the difficult times we go through into our bodies, responding to emotional stress with physical tension, especially in the shoulder and neck muscles. And from an early age we prepare ourselves for back problems with a posture fault which is almost universal: walking with feet angled outwards, the back hollowed and the stomach out.

It's an adult version of the nursery stagger we all did when we were in nappies, and which most of us go on doing for ever after.

As we grow older, the shoulders tend to slump forward, compressing the rib-cage and pushing the upper part of the torso downwards. As a result, the waist thickens, the shoulder and neck muscles tighten, and the 'dowager's hump' and double chin make their appearance.

Gradually our muscles and tendons stretch or shorten to accommodate our bad body position and we are unaware of the damage it is causing. This collapse downwards inhibits our movements and prepares the way for stiff joints, backache, arthritis, nervous tension, headaches and more. (Don't go away, there is a happy ending!)

When you suffer from an aching back or stiff knees you naturally look for a remedy for that particular problem. But if this stiffness or pain is caused by poor alignment the long-term cure lies in improving the way you co-ordinate every part of yourself.

Men and women of all ages and occupations come to me for help: teenagers with hunched shoulders and curved spines trying to hide their height; dentists with stiff shoulders and necks; pregnant women with aching backs and feet; pianists with arthritic wrists; people with all kinds of back problems.

How this book can help

One of the most important parts of this book is at the beginning of Section I where I show you how to 'touch learn' your joints and muscles so that you can see how they relate to each other. Don't skip it. It is vital to understand how your body works both intellectually and through the actual physical sense of the parts moving and relating to each other.

Using this Touch Knowledge as the foundation, you will be taught to do the three basic alignments: the standing, the sitting and the lying-down. These, with their Releases and Stretches, form exercise units called 3-Sets and should be practised daily.

Doing this, plus the everyday applications shown in Section II, will help re-educate your joints and muscles into their new positions. Simple daily activities such as talking on the telephone, driving a car, going up and down stairs will strengthen your muscles so that in time you will not have consciously to re-align your body so often.

Re-alignment starts with those long-suffering, battered appendages we call our feet – the most neglected parts of the human body. Many people have problems with their feet because they stand and walk with the body weight on the big-toe joint. The strain of the weight enlarges the toe joint and at the same time flattens the arches and weakens the ankles. The joints of all the toes are vital in helping to support your weight. I shall teach you how to stand on your feet correctly so that the body weight is supported by the entire foot. It is essential to get the feet correct before you begin to attempt to align the rest of your body.

If you have to stand or walk for any length of time, your weight will not hammer your feet into the ground. The upward thrust of your body will take the downward pressure of your weight off your feet. Walking will become a well co-ordinated pleasure. You will have lightened the burden by literally taking the weight off your feet.

Long-term benefits to look forward to

The benefits are immeasurable. Correcting the overall collapse of the body frees the internal organs from compression so that they can function more efficiently. You will have renewed energy because re-alignment will correct all the debilitating things you were doing with your body.

In the long term, correct alignment will

- Reduce enlarged joints of the feet
- Raise your arches
- Improve circulation
- Help alleviate arthritis, rheumatism and headaches
- Strengthen weak ankles
- Keep joints flexible
- Stretch your hamstrings

— Help correct lower-back problems
— Improve breathing
— Improve digestion
— Relieve tension

Knowing that you have a simple, precise technique for removing tension at any time puts you in control. Since how your body feels instantly affects how *you* feel, that control will give you a sense of achievement which will do wonders for your self-confidence.

I am not suggesting that you should walk tall and sit straight every moment of the day. That's no way to win friends and influence people. When you want to relax, relax. That's OK. Allowing any exercise discipline to rule your life to the exclusion of all else is as bad as never doing any exercise at all.

Life is a balancing act. Moderation is what sustains us all. This work is about being flexible and keeping your options open. Once you know the techniques you will be free to choose whether you want to sit up straight or relax. The difference is that, whereas before you slumped, now you will relax. Slumping causes muscle tension and strain. Relaxation releases tension.

Just in case I have given you the teeniest impression that, like Dr Beecham's pills, re-alignment will cure just about everything – it won't. But it *will* help you face whatever challenges life has in store. If you do fall flat on your face (and who doesn't at some time?), you will pick yourself up faster and more easily. You will be more resilient. Being flexible in body and mind means that you won't *break* so easily.

You will smile more often – both because you feel good and because correct alignment actually lifts up your 'smiling' muscles. Life will be more fun.

I should have called this 'A Serious Book on How to Smile' because that is what it is all about.

So, please, don't just read it. Do it.

GETTING IT STRAIGHT

GETTING READY TO START LEARNING HOW

In most books that fall under the heading of instruction, especially self-instruction, there is some isolated chapter, usually at the beginning, on how to use the book. I have always found this a bit frustrating. What I always want is to have the advice on 'how to' ready at hand as I am reading the book. In the hope that you feel the same, this is the way *this* book has been written. As you read, and do, the advice will be there. Please do not skip – things won't work if you do. The first thing we must find out is where we are going to put ourselves to start the big change; so, some words on

Location

In the early days of learning how to re-align your body, using the book as a guide, I would advise you to find a place where you can work alone. You will be adjusting your body with your hands in order to understand how it is hinged together, and doing things that are quite new and different. All in all, it is better at this point to avoid having to deal with 'What *are* you doing?' questions. Your private place does not have to be large; you need just enough space to stand up, extend your arms to the side, and lie down, and it would help if there were enough room to give yourself a little walkaround between attempts.

Equipment

You certainly do not need much equipment. Just make sure that whatever you are standing or sitting on cannot move about. Small rugs on slippery floors do not make for a firm footing under any conditions. Also, do not work on deep-pile carpets or rugs where you sink in to your knees. Flat floors or flat carpets are definitely best.

You'll need a space of wall you can lean against while sitting on the floor.

If a window comes under the heading of equipment, it would be nice to have one. Remember, you will be using your body and thinking about what you are doing. Both of these profit from a little fresh air. One real must for the sitting alignment is a chair – an old-fashioned straight chair with no arms that everyone used to have around and has probably thrown out. No slanted seats, please.

Clothes

While you are in the learning stage, you should wear as little as possible or, more accurately, clothes that enable you to move your body easily, let you touch and feel the various parts, and do not obscure your shape. For example, leotards and tights are good, but a track-suit is not; bathing-trunks and a vest are fine but long-johns fall somewhere in between; nudity tends to distract. But one thing *is* a must: bare feet throughout the learning period, please.

The best way of learning the instructions

At this point, let us try to overcome one incontrovertible problem; reading something that requires you to follow instructions with your body at the same time is not easy, and I would like to suggest a means of working with this book that will help to solve this problem and bring with it a very useful bonus. I am reluctant to ask you to buy anything unless I feel it will definitely improve the effectiveness of the teaching. In this case it will, so I strongly suggest that, if you do not own an audio-tape recorder, please think seriously about borrowing one.

Here is the programme I recommend for maximum effectiveness in learning from this book, starting with the chapter called 'The Touch Knowledge of Your Body'.

FIRST, READ THE CHAPTER THROUGH TO YOURSELF

This will provide an understanding in your head, before your head and body have to work together.

SECOND, RECORD YOURSELF READING THE CHAPTER

Do this at a tempo you find personally satisfactory, but keep it fairly slow, as you will need time to co-ordinate your movements with the instructions. You may, if you wish, put in asides that have occurred to you while you were reading the chapter to yourself – words of your own that may aid you in the execution.

THEN – DO THE CHAPTER WHILE YOU LISTEN TO YOUR RECORDING

This way, you will not have to interrupt the continuity of movement in order to read what comes next. You can stop the tape whenever you wish to take a look at the text or the illustrations, or repeat some movement that needs further experimentation. It is possible to do these things, resume the recording and move on to the next step. The added bonus is that this method provides you with your own personal 'voice-over': you will be telling yourself what to do, using my instructions. It sets the tone for an important factor in the success of the alignment concept – you will be assuming a greater responsibility for getting it straight.

I suggest you start recording your voice on the Touch Knowledge. When you see how it goes you may want to use it on all the chapters: I shall suggest you do so where I think it will be helpful.

Mirrors – yes or no?
Mostly no. Like nudity, they tend to distract. In the process of peering into them, you risk disturbing what you have already aligned. Also, you can't carry them about with you. Use them to check certain things only, then when you are satisfied close

your eyes to get the *feel*. The feel you *can* carry with you. In certain parts of the book I shall help you to learn to do this.

Remember, a mirror is not you. It is just a reflection. *You* create the real image.

About breathing

This is a subject on which volumes have been written – almost every one contradicting the next. Since it is my view that life, and living it, should be approached with workable practicality, here are my workable, practical suggestions on breathing.

1. Ideally, you should breathe through the nose. That is what it is for. It is beautifully designed for the purpose, having a nice funnel-like shape and tiny hairs on the inside that help to filter out pollution and warm the air as it comes in.
2. Ideally, you should start body movements downwards with an exhale, and movements upwards with an inhale. This coincides with emptying and filling the lungs, useful to remember when putting down or picking up objects.
3. On the subject of lungs, they work better if you open up the area in which they have to operate. Common sense tells you that hunching your shoulders forward collapses and lessens the space the lungs have to work in, and inhibits their ability to function efficiently. The re-structured alignment will teach you how to correct this, so that in movement or non-movement you will be able to feed in more air.
4. In general, use your own natural breathing rhythm. Because it is automatic and unconscious you will not have to give it any additional consideration. It is easier to maintain and integrate into movement.

Above all, TRY NOT TO STOP! Even suspending your breath temporarily, as we do sometimes when concentrating, makes you short of breath. Keep it going.

You are ready to start reading the Touch Knowledge.

THE TOUCH KNOWLEDGE OF YOUR BODY

Getting to know yourself

Correct alignment means co-ordinating every part of your body in its correct relationship to the other parts. Knowing how to do this requires not only that you understand the instructions, but also that you *feel* how to do it with your body.

You will learn, by touch, the relationship of one part of your body to another, working primarily through the skeletal structure. The aim is to learn to *feel* how one part of your body affects another.

Set some time aside for yourself. Ideally the Touch Knowledge should be carried out in one continuous session. But if tiredness or circumstances make this impracticable, then make the break at the mid-point of the instructions (page 36).

Many people regard their body as if it were somehow forbidden territory. Well, we're going to change all that. These touch exercises are designed to enable you and your body to get to know each other.

It is *your* body and as owner-occupier you should be familiar with the working layout and look on it as something which needs regular maintenance to keep it running smoothly. You can't ever really *stop* exercising, just moving about from day to day, but the thing to control is whether you are exercising to benefit or to harm.

Please read this whole chapter through before you do any of it, as I have advised. Record yourself reading it. Then listen to the recording as you follow the instructions.

The feet

Sit on the floor with your back against a flat wall and your legs straight out in front of you. (The end of a sofa or anything which is vertical and stable enough for you to lean against will do, but a wall does the job better.) Check that your bottom is fairly close to the wall.

Now flex your right knee and place your right foot flat on the floor. Check that your foot is straight, not angled inwards or outwards, and close enough to put both hands on it; see that your right knee is in a straight line with your right ankle. (Extend your left leg somewhat to the side in a position that is comfortable.)

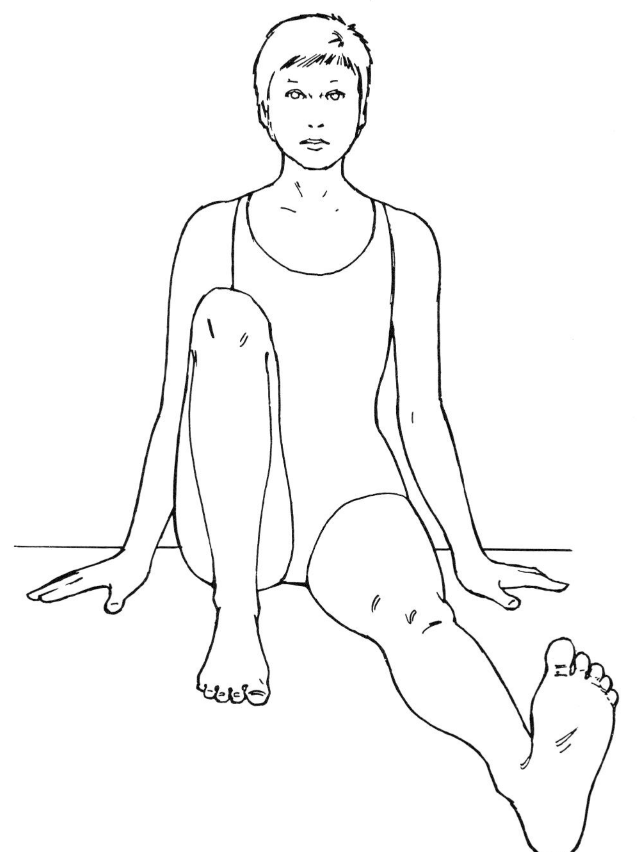

You are going to examine your right foot by touch, starting with the toes. With your right thumb, find the joint that joins the big toe to the foot. The sketch will give you a general idea but the exact location varies with the individual. Keep your thumb on this joint and with your forefinger pull up the end of your toe. Hold it for a moment and feel the stretch.

Since we seldom stretch our toes, the tendons are reluctant to co-operate and you'll find the rest of your toes joining the big toe in this upward movement. Make them wait their turn and try to keep them on the ground as much as possible, because you want to feel the stretch in each toe individually. Place your big toe back on the ground, pointing straight ahead.

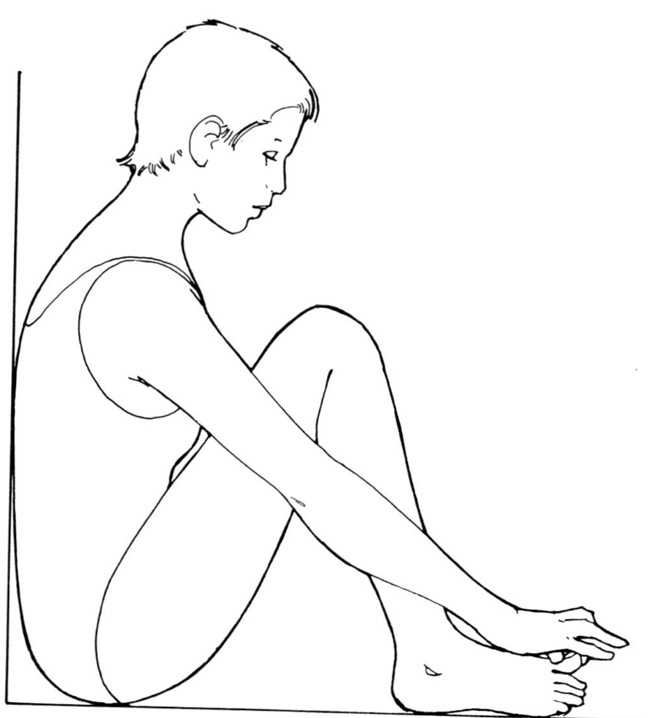

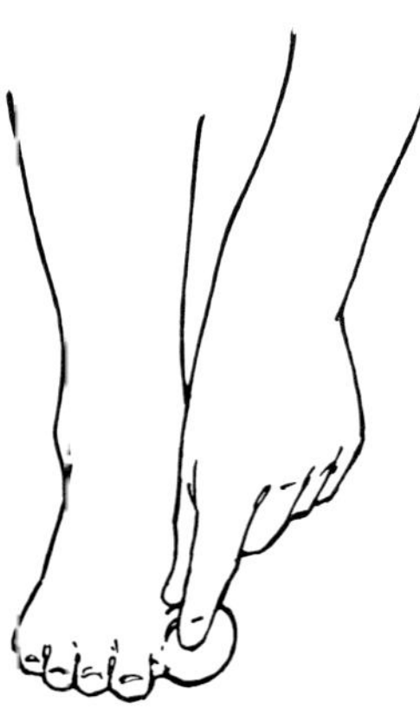

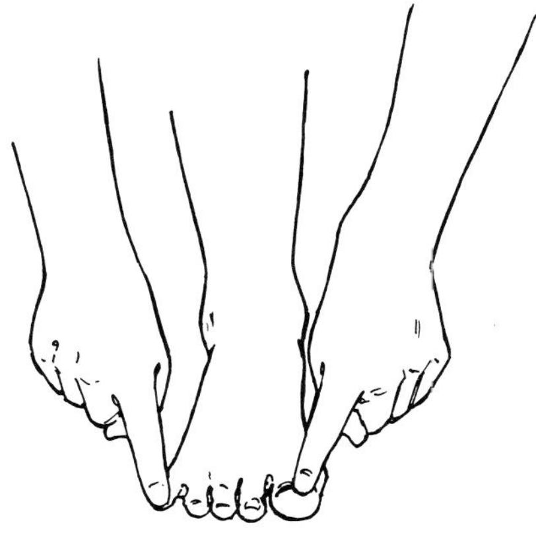

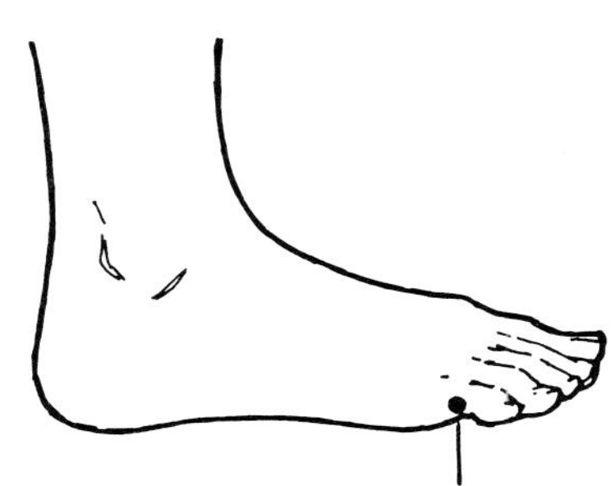

Move on to your second, third and fourth toes. Find the joint of each one with your thumb and lift each toe upwards with your forefinger as you did with the big toe. They'll probably feel increasingly stiff as you move towards the little toe. This is caused by years of being pushed close together in shoes.

Now for your little toe – neglected and unused and therefore probably quite numb. Find the joint with your thumb and lift the toe as you did the others.

Put your left index finger on your right big toe with enough pressure to keep it pointing straight forward. At the same time, with the right hand, pull your little toe away from the others as far as it will go.

You should feel a stretch across the joints from the big to the little toe. Now place your little toe flat on the floor, letting it keep its distance from the other toes if you can.

On the outside of the little-toe joint you'll find a soft spot. Use the sketch as a guide but, again, the exact position varies slightly with the individual.

With your right forefinger, move this soft spot down to the floor so that you can actually see, with the movement, the outside of your foot going down in closer contact with the floor.

When your little toe is stretched out and brought down it will begin to affect the entire balance of the foot.

The ankles

The result of walking and standing with the feet angled outwards, however slightly, is that the weight enlarges the big-toe joint, flattens the arches and weakens the ankles, which are gradually pushed inwards.

With the feet straight and the little toe brought down we can begin to move the ankles back to where they should be – neither pushed inwards nor outwards. (See top of next page.)

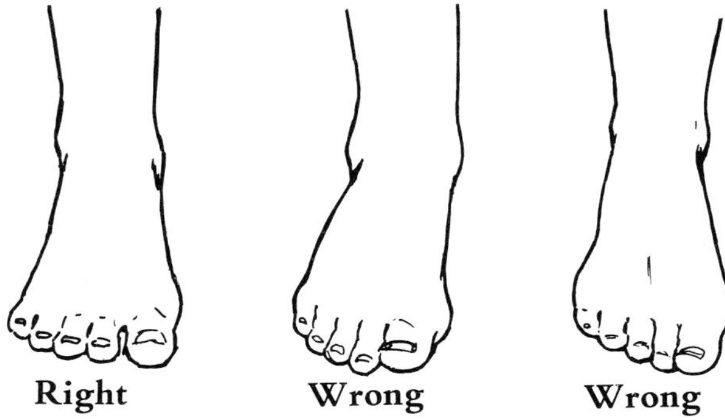

Move your right hand along the outer edge of your right foot (it should now be so firmly on the floor that you cannot get your fingers underneath it) until you arrive just in front of the projecting ankle bone. Move your fingers up towards the front of the ankle bone, pressing gently as you go, until you find a soft, possibly sensitive hollow and leave your fingers pressed into that hollow.

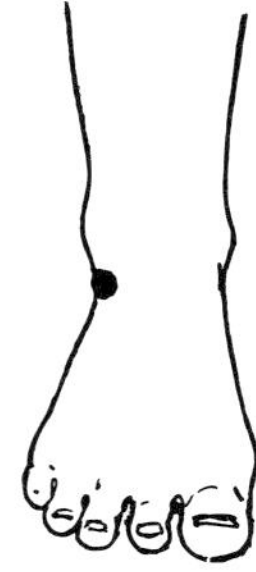

With your left hand find the opposite hollow on the *inside* of your right ankle. Slide your index finger about half an inch down until you find a projecting bone. Keeping your finger on this bone and pushing it inwards, roll your foot very slightly towards the outside. Do not overdo this, as you do not want to twist your ankle to the outside. Stop when you see, and can feel with your fingers, that there is an *even* and *equal* placement of the hollows under each side of your ankle bones.

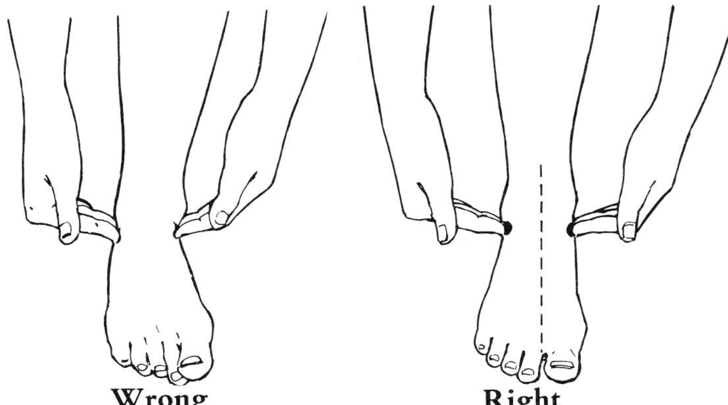

Try to keep your knee joint in line over the ankle while you are doing this; you'll find it helps to keep your foot in place. Take your time and keep experimenting with this ankle adjustment, moving from the incorrect to the correct position until you understand and feel it exactly.

A word of encouragement: don't be dismayed if you think you are not getting it right first time. Take each stage slowly and easily and enjoy feeling your body move under your hands.

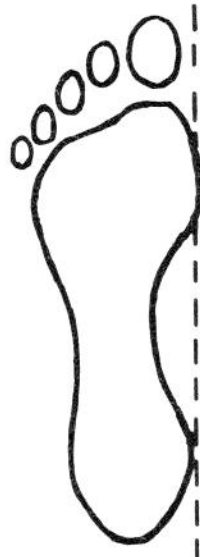

Now move your hands from your ankle to your heel and run your thumbs down the back of the heel to the floor. (Getting to know the feel of the heels when they are pushed down to the floor will help you know how and where they are when we use them later on.) You should now be able to 'sketch' a straight line from your big-toe joint to the inner side of your heel. If you move your hands along the inside and outside of your foot towards the toes, you'll feel how your arch has been raised and the outer edge of your foot has been brought down into contact with the floor. It is the little-toe stretch and ankle adjustment which raise the arch and take the weight off the joint of the big toe.

Finally, stroke each toe in turn with the tip of your index finger, gently flattening the length of the toe into the floor from the base of each joint to the toe-nail, with the big toe straight forward and the little toe to the side.

This is the foot position on which you are going to build your new alignment.

Now stretch your right leg out on the floor, bring up your left foot close to your buttocks and go through the same process with your left foot.

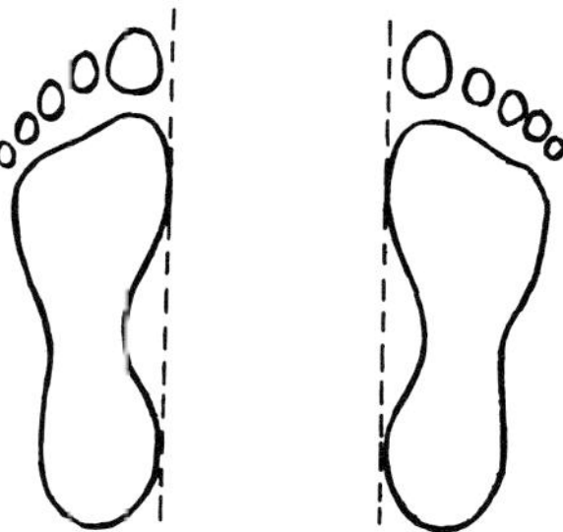

The centre of the ankle joints

Bring your right foot up to join your left. The feet should be placed about six inches apart, be parallel and, as well as you are able, in the final corrected position you have achieved by working with your toe and ankle joints.

Throughout the next and ensuing movements please try to ensure that your knees also remain six inches apart.

Place your thumbs on the soft centres of your ankle joints – between the projecting bones, the ankle condyles, that jut out on either side.

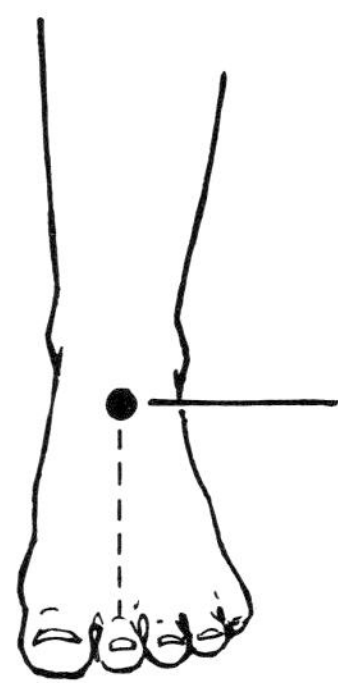

You are about to define the line of balance over the instep. With your foot in the corrected position, leave your thumbs in place in those soft hollows and place your forefingers in the space between your big and second toes. This line, from ankle to toe over the instep, defines the place over which your body will be balanced.

Whenever I say, 'Be sure that your weight is over your instep,' that is the place I mean. If your ankles are slanted inwards or twisted outwards, that line of balance is going to be disturbed.

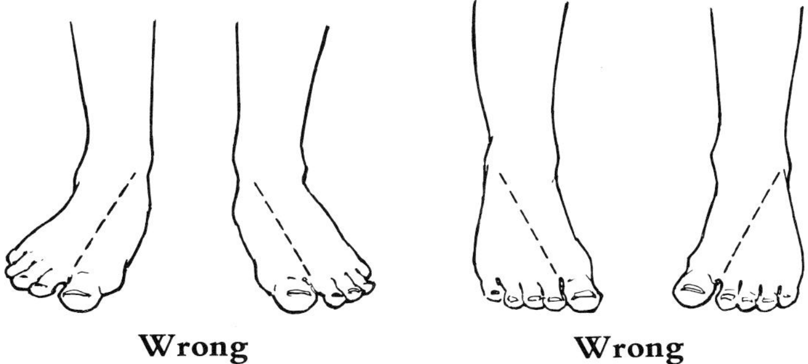

The knees

Now that you've seen how the placement of your foot affects the position of your ankle, I will show you how the position of the ankle affects that of your knees.

Cup your right hand around your right ankle, and your left hand round the left one, and move both hands up along your shin bones to your knee-caps. On the outside of each knee-cap you'll find another soft depression. Place your hands along the outsides so that your middle fingers can push into soft depressions, and leave them there.

Now let's experiment. Move your feet out of line – so that they slant outwards instead of being straight and parallel – and push your ankles inwards. You should be able to feel a corresponding movement in that area of the knee joint.

Now go back to the correct placement of the feet – straight and parallel – and you should feel the centre of each knee-cap move so that it is in line with the centre of the ankle. This line-up lessens the pressure on these joints and helps them support each other.

Finally, direct the knee-caps slightly inwards (not pushed together, but directed towards a centre point). This slight

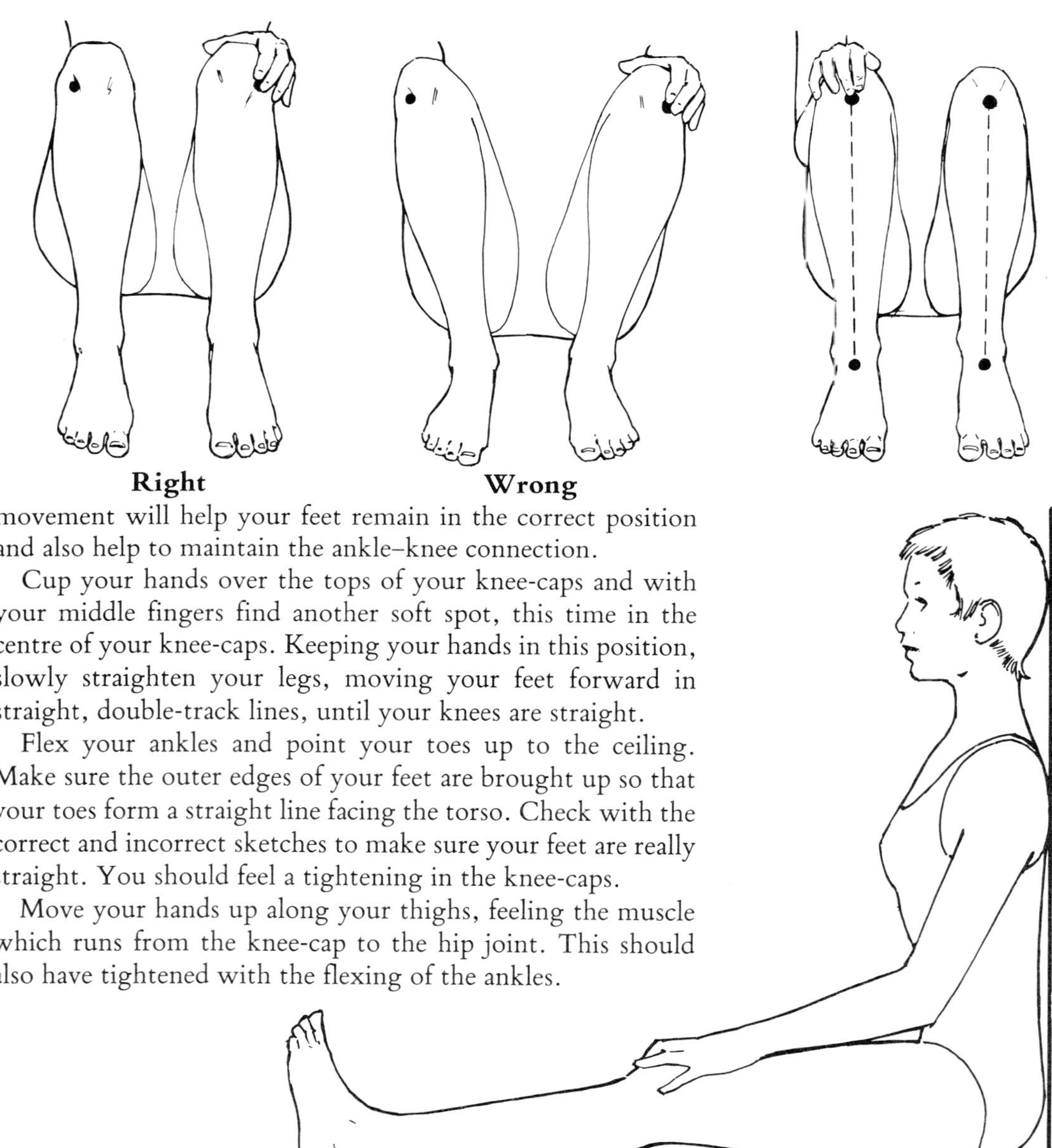

movement will help your feet remain in the correct position and also help to maintain the ankle–knee connection.

Cup your hands over the tops of your knee-caps and with your middle fingers find another soft spot, this time in the centre of your knee-caps. Keeping your hands in this position, slowly straighten your legs, moving your feet forward in straight, double-track lines, until your knees are straight.

Flex your ankles and point your toes up to the ceiling. Make sure the outer edges of your feet are brought up so that your toes form a straight line facing the torso. Check with the correct and incorrect sketches to make sure your feet are really straight. You should feel a tightening in the knee-caps.

Move your hands up along your thighs, feeling the muscle which runs from the knee-cap to the hip joint. This should also have tightened with the flexing of the ankles.

Reach behind and probe your right buttock to locate the solid bone-end embedded there. Find it, and for ever after let's call it the 'sitting bone'.

Grasp the right 'sitting bone' from underneath and move it, and your buttock with it, back to the wall as far as it will go. Remove your hand and get that buttock cheek well settled on the floor.

If you have done this successfully, your right leg will now appear shorter than your left. Remedy this by doing exactly the same with your left buttock. Now you will have two shorter legs and a much straighter back.

If, while doing this, your feet and legs have moved out of line, re-align them into the correct position before continuing.

If your hamstrings (along the back of your legs) are causing

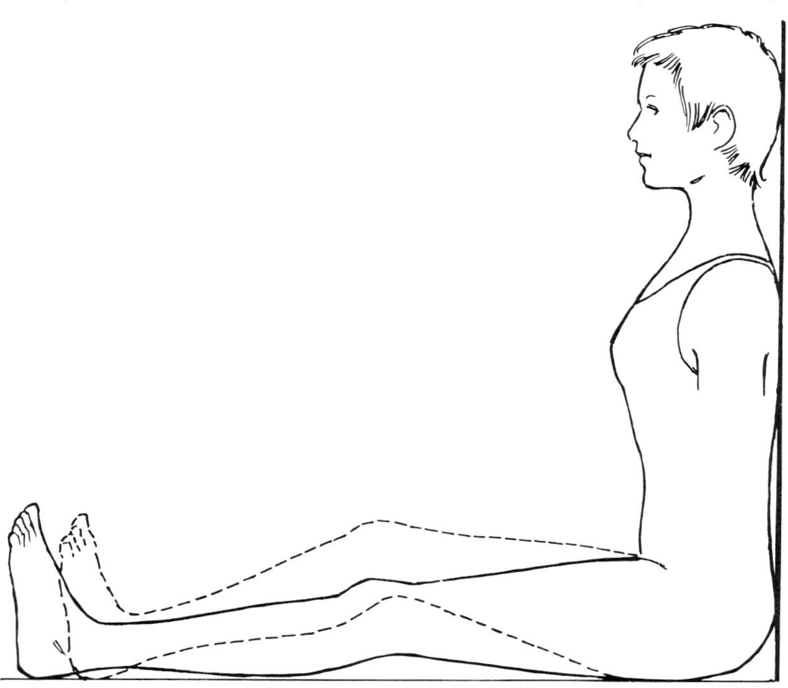

discomfort, you may flex your knees a little. Now you will begin to understand why, if you stand, walk, run or do anything with your feet splayed, your knees probably are never completely straightened and in turn your hamstrings never really stretched.

If you have to flex your knees for comfort, check that the centres of your knee-caps are still in line with the centres of your ankles, and watch that your feet remain in their parallel corrected position.

Using both hands, separate the cheeks of your buttocks by rocking from side to side. Make sure the buttocks are relaxed, not tense. Tightened buttocks open the front of the pelvis outwards and stretch the abdominal muscles outwards too. This causes the stomach to stick out (because it has no support) and the lower back to curve in.

Hip rotation

The effect of this movement is a continuous tightening along the upper thighs into the abdominal muscles. I'd like you to do it first incorrectly and then correctly, so that you can register the difference.

Check that your hips are well back under your torso. If you have flexed your knees, straighten them. Find the ball-and-

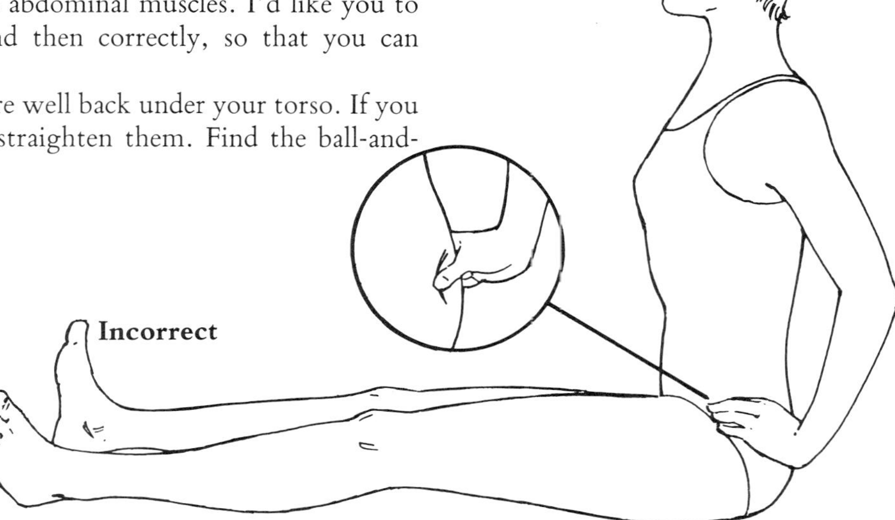

Incorrect

socket joint where the thigh bone moves in the pelvis. Put your thumbs behind on these hip joints and your fingers forward into your groin.

To achieve the *incorrect* position, allow your feet to fall apart in an exaggerated angle outwards. Notice how your knees flex immediately and how you can feel in your fingertips that the area in front of your hip joints spreads and loosens. The abdominal muscles loosen because the pelvis opens outwards in this position. This also happens when you are standing with your feet angled outwards, creating a protruding, dropped stomach and a sway back.

Now, to achieve the *correct* position, move your feet back into the straight, parallel position. Lift your toes and point them straight up towards the ceiling and push your heels away from the torso. Direct your knees slightly inwards. Don't raise your heels.

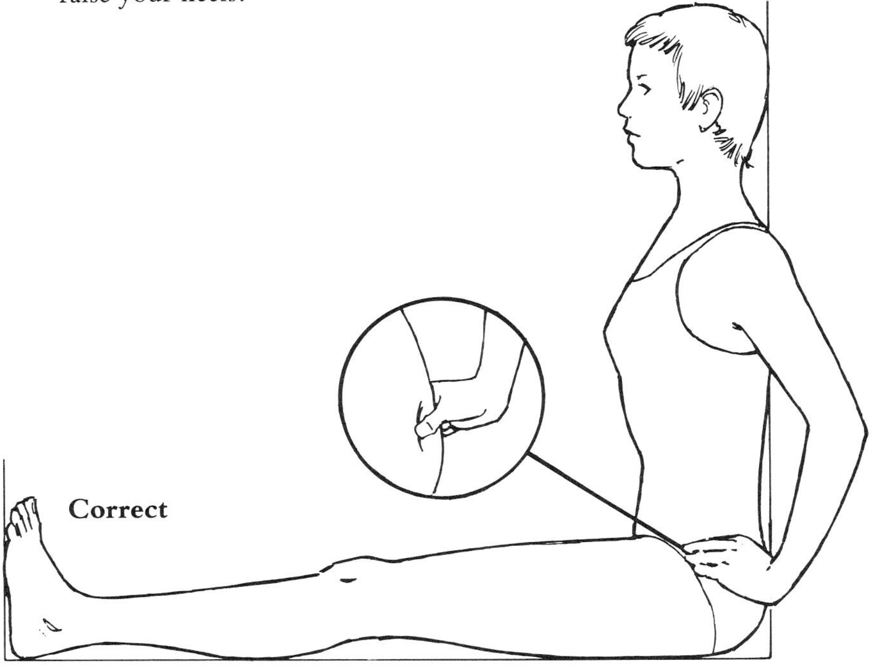

Correct

You should see a tightening of the knees and upper thighs and, most important of all, feel under your forefingers a pull of muscle into the centre of your abdomen. Exaggerate the movement until you can feel this with your fingers.

Move your feet from the incorrect position (an exaggerated outward angle) back to the correct position (straight and parallel) several times to feel the difference. The correct way is how you achieve a flat stomach, sitting, standing or lying down.

If it is necessary for you to do this let-your-fingers-do-the-walking of the body in two stages, this is the time to take a break.

The next stage will be done sitting in the straight chair and, although you've moved from the floor up to the chair, we are going to get the lower half of your body into a position comparable to that which you achieved sitting on the floor.

Sit on the chair so that the two 'sitting bones' in your buttocks are brought forward to the edge of the chair, with your feet flat on the floor in their corrected position about six inches apart (toes straight forward and ankles 'even and equal'), your knees flexed with the knee-caps directly above the centre of the ankles and directed *slightly* inwards.

The spine

Place your hands on the outside of your buttocks. Rock slightly from side to side while pulling outwards with your hands so that those two big 'sitting bones' are spread apart.

Now move your RIGHT hand behind you and place it, palm down, on your lower back just above the buttocks. With your middle finger reach down and place it on your coccyx – the very end of your spinal column, between the cheeks of your buttocks.

Bring your LEFT hand round in front of your torso and place it, palm down, between the hip joints, just above the pubis. With the middle finger of your right hand, push the coccyx firmly downwards and towards the seat of the chair.

You should feel with this movement a tightening UP and IN of the lower abdominal muscles.

Move your right hand slowly up your spine. Locate each vertebra separately and push it firmly inwards. Simultaneously move your left hand up the front of your torso, feeling an upward stretch of the muscles.

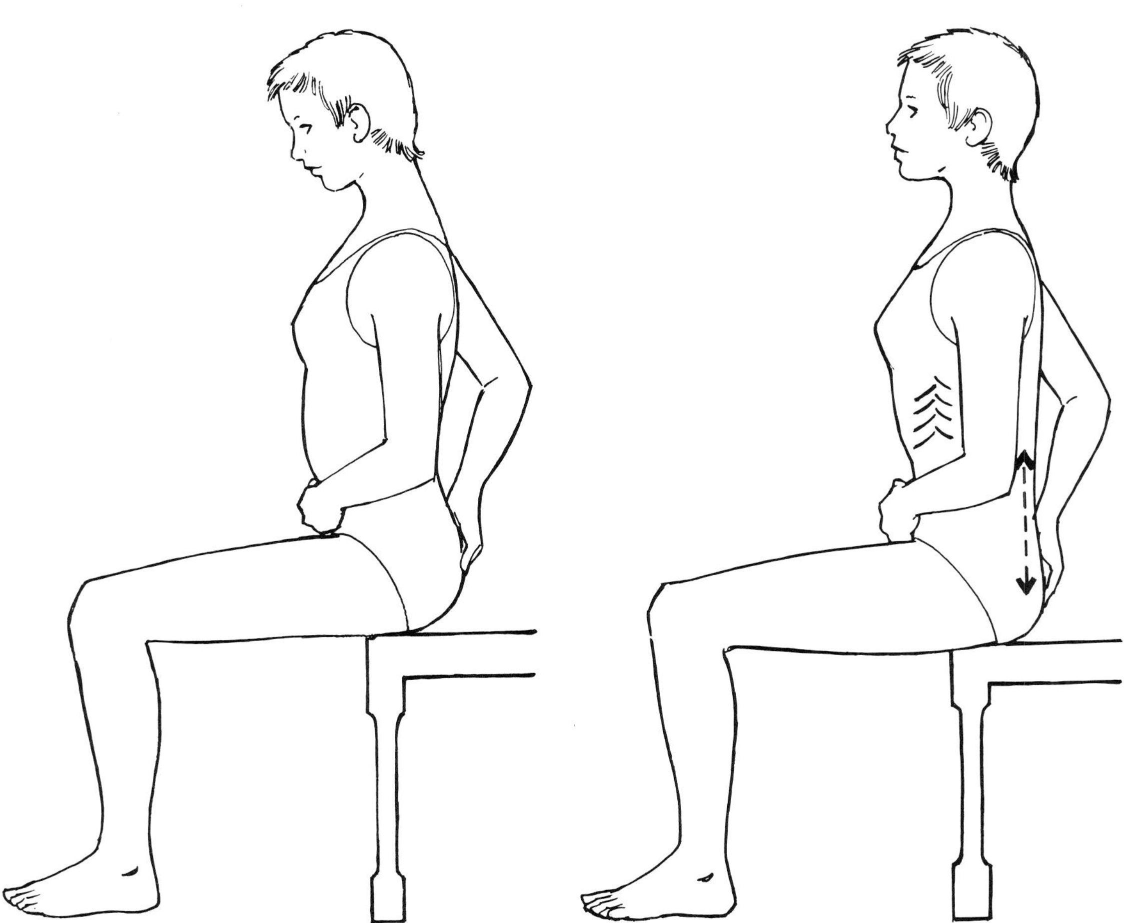

At this point in your intense concentration for goodness sake don't forget to keep breathing!

When you get about two-thirds of the way up your spine, which is about as far as you can reach, pause. Your left hand should then be just under the bottom of your rib-cage. Push the vertebra you're touching with your right hand firmly inwards and with your left hand you will be able to feel your rib-cage lifting.

Throughout this spinal stretch, try to keep your coccyx well down and to hold the tightening of the abdomen 'up and in', so that you don't curve the lower back.

Now move your hands to the front and place them over the two 'wings' of the rib-cage, with the fingertips almost touching.

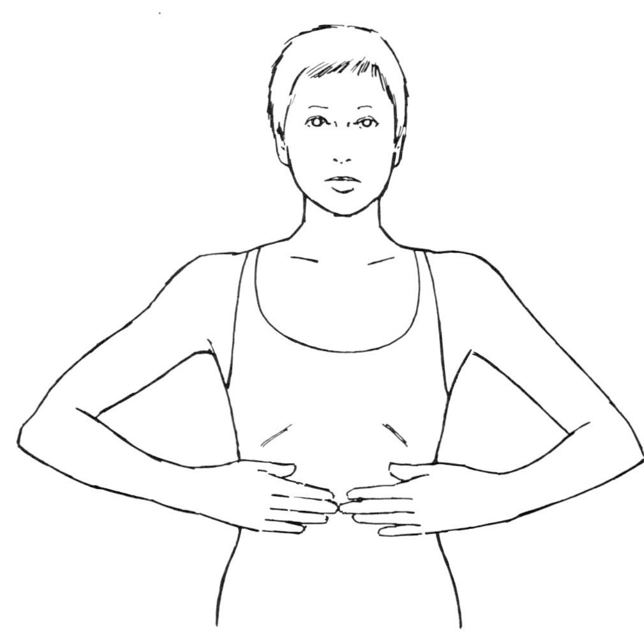

Move your fingers up the centre of the chest, between the breasts, to the point of the neck. Along this line you will feel a fine mesh of bone, quite sensitive and compressed in places. That is because, with the shoulders forward, it *is* compressed.

When your fingers reach the little hollow at the base of your neck, move your hands apart, one to the left, the other to the right, across your collar bone to the tips of your shoulders. These are rotating ball-and-socket joints. Try to span them with your fingers in front and thumbs behind. It's not so easy with stiff joints, but do the best you can.

Ideally, your elbows should be along the side of your torso but you will probably have to angle them out a little at this stage.

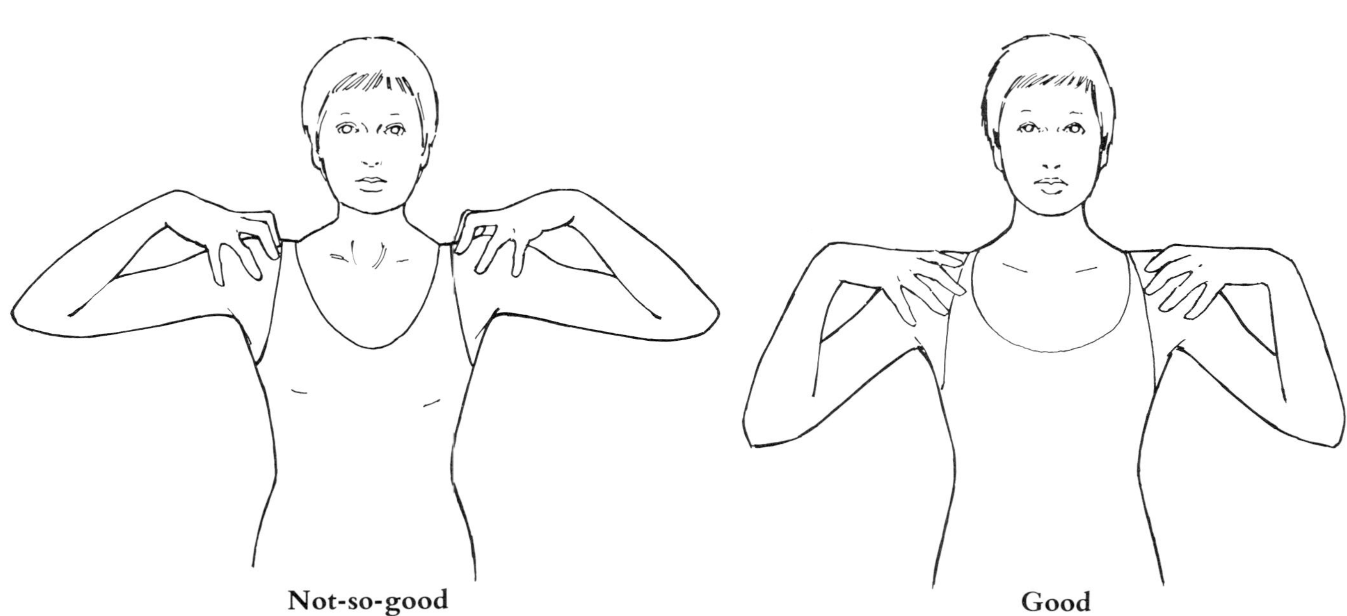

Not-so-good **Good**

The shoulder rotation
We are now going to learn a rotation of the shoulders away from the debilitating shoulder-curved-forward posture.

With your hands still spanning your shoulder joints, raise your shoulders up towards your ears half an inch, then move them back towards your spine half an inch, and then pull them straight down one inch. As you bring your shoulders down you should be able to move your elbows closer into and alongside your torso.

This shoulder rotation helps hold the shoulders down into their sockets, flattens the back muscles, pulls in the shoulder blades, raises the breastbone and altogether reinforces the straightening of the spine.

Make sure you do not rotate the shoulders full circle and simply go back to the original position. The rotation is a half circle: up, back and down. The more round-shouldered you've been, the more trouble you'll have doing this.

Keep practising! We're not looking for perfection, but the more you do it the easier it will become.

The arms and hands
Stretch your right arm straight in front of you, palm upwards. Make a fist. Bring the fist up towards your shoulder by flexing and lowering the elbow. Keep the fist in front of and in line with your shoulder, and stop when it is about six inches away from your shoulder joint.

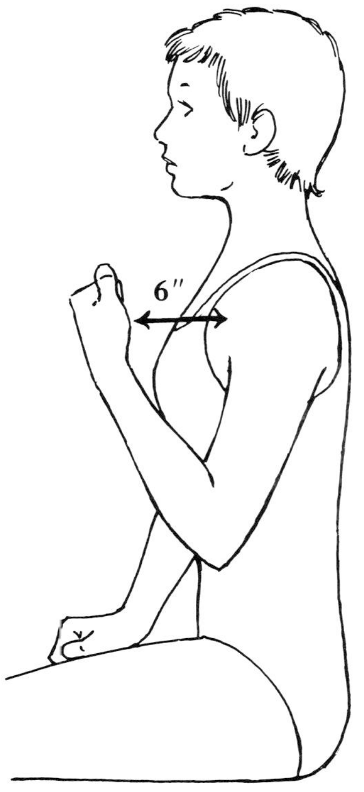

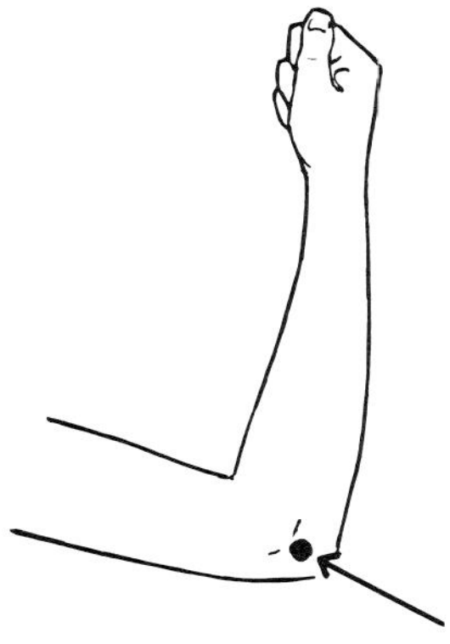

With your left hand locate the soft part below the outside protrusion of your right elbow joint, just as you did with the soft spot in the knee joint. Hold on to this soft area and straighten your elbow so that your fist is extended in front of you.

Now open your fist and straighten your fingers so that they stay together (including the little finger and thumb) and extend them directly forward. As you stretch them you should feel the elbow tighten. The stronger the stretch, the more it affects the joint.

Now turn your extended hand over so that your palm is facing inwards. Take your left hand away. Keeping your right arm straight from shoulder to fingertips, drop it straight down until it is in a straight line alongside your torso. Remember the elbow, wrist and fingers stay straight and the arm finishes with the fingertips together and pointing directly to the ground.

Because in this movement you will probably have disturbed your shoulder rotation placement, repeat it once more: leaving your arm alongside the torso, palm facing in, raise your shoulder half an inch, back half an inch, then down one inch. Now really straighten your elbow, wrist and fingertips. As you will feel, this helps to hold your shoulder in its correct position. Now repeat everything with your left arm.

When you have finished, position yourself with both arms straight down alongside your torso. As you stretch your fingertips towards the floor, you should feel a tightening pull in the back muscles behind the shoulder joints.

Take a breath, exhale, and have courage – we're on our way to the finishing post.

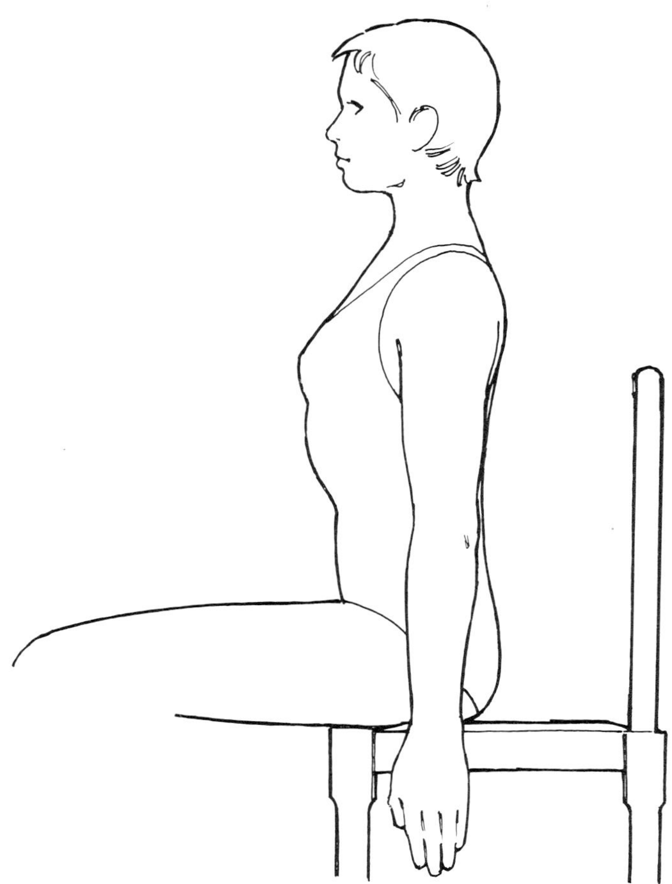

The neck and head

Put both hands behind the base of your neck, with your fingers touching, and move your fingers up the back of your neck until they reach the hollow just below your skull.

Move both hands up to the crown of your head. Bring your elbows to the front so that your forearms are roughly parallel, and keep your shoulders down as you move your hands over

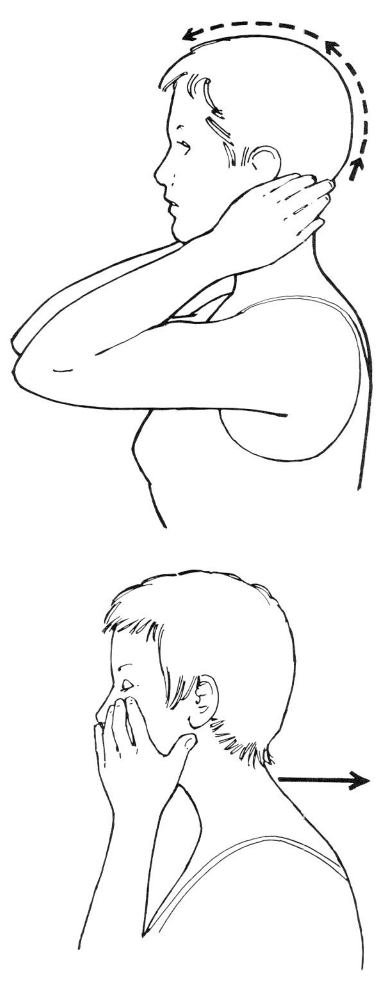

the crown and down the centre of your forehead. Keep your middle fingers together and move them down between your eyebrows. Separate your fingers and run the middle finger of each hand down the sides of your nose until they rest alongside the nostrils – but don't press!

Leaving your fingers there, extend your thumbs and place them just below the chin line. With your right thumb to the right, and your left to the left, feel along that bone until your thumbs are fitted behind the hinges of your jaw. At this point check that your shoulders are down and that your chin is not lowered.

Keeping your thumbs in these hinges, push your head back as far as it will go towards your spine. Keep your eyes straight forward and do not lift or lower your chin. You should feel the space behind your jaw hinge closing.

To check that you have got this very important movement correct, exaggerate the wrong position by pushing your chin forward as far as it will go. Feel the space behind the jaw hinge, just in front of the ear lobes. Now push your head back as far as it will go towards your spine, and feel your jaw hinge move back and the space close.

Big breath. Exhale. Let go – now you can relax.

Congratulations!

You have completed the Touch Knowledge of your body. It will equip you to use your body with more than superficial awareness and it is vital to what we are going to do together. The correct inter-relationship of the parts is the basis for 'getting it straight' and it will always, as we work together, be observed.

You won't be required to do this again, but my suggestion – and it is something I do – is to use it to counteract those times when you seem to have lost touch with yourself. It is a very positive, tactile process and puts you securely in the role of owner-occupier.

AFTER THE TOUCH KNOWLEDGE

We are now going to take what you have learned about body logic (i.e. how one part affects the others) and apply it to learning to align your body correctly in the standing, sitting and lying positions. These are the three basic body positions assumed in daily living. I am also going to give you two additional things to do with these re-structured positions to create a more balanced alignment programme. These are called Releases and Stretches. They are simply wonderful to do and will help both in implementing the alignment concept and in strengthening the muscles you'll need in order to be at ease in the alignment. Mind you, they will not, just as everything else in this book will not, contradict the basic alignment rules. For easy reference, from now on we shall refer to the Alignment, the Release and the Stretch as a 3-Set.

It is a good idea to go into the Standing 3-Set lesson fairly shortly after you do the Touch Knowledge, while the awareness is still bubbling. Go back to your private place not more than one or two days later, unless of course you simply cannot manage it. In that case, either read the Touch Knowledge again or, if you've recorded yourself on this chapter, listen to it.

Just one more point: I use the word 'flex' to describe the joints creating an angled line. It seems more accurate than 'bend'.

THE STANDING 3-SET

The alignment

This is a series of simple movements which will enable you to straighten your body from the feet upwards and co-ordinate every one of your joints and muscles in its correct relationship to the others. These movements are all inter-related. You must maintain each new position as you move on to the next, otherwise you will throw out of line whatever you have already accomplished.

The release

This is a series of movements that enables you to transform the strongly held vertical line of the aligned body into a self-supported curve. For flexibility the spine must be exercised from time to time in a curved position. In this position it is protected from strain by support of the elbows. But please note that *no other exercise in this book should be done with your back in a curved position*.

The abdominal muscles can be pulled really high up so they can be tightened to the maximum. The weight of the head is taken on the fists which, coupled with the bringing down of the shoulders, relieves tension in the neck. The rocking movement is ancient, primal and wonderfully soothing; as a big bonus, it keeps your balancing act going better.

The stretch

The stretch is a series of movements that enables you to return your body to a vertically aligned position and then to stretch your muscles and use your breathing to release concentrated energy.

HOW TO DO IT

The first practical step towards re-alignment is to learn a new way of standing on your own feet. Most people angle their feet slightly, and sometimes markedly, outwards, so their weight puts a strain on the big-toe joints, which eventually enlarge under that strain. This angled position of the feet also flattens the arches, weakens the ankles and has a debilitating effect on the entire alignment of the body.

Stand up and look down at your feet. Move them about six to ten inches apart in parallel lines. Never work with your feet farther apart than the outside line of the feet in line with the outside of the hips, otherwise your weight distribution will be affected and you will not be well balanced. Check that your big toes are facing directly forward.

Remembering how the joints of each toe felt in the Touch Knowledge exercise, lift all your toes upwards towards the ceiling, keeping the balls of your feet on the floor. Try not to rock back on your heels. Bring all the toes up to more or less the same height.

Keeping your big toes straight forward, stretch all your other toes apart, extending the little toes as far as possible out to the sides.

Now place all your toes down flat on the floor, still stretched. Check that your big toes are still directed forward and that the little toes have stretched and are in contact with the floor.

Most people stand with their ankles in a position that pushes their weight on to the inside of the feet instead of being evenly distributed.

In order to use the outside of the foot sufficiently to achieve an 'even and equal' weight distribution you must make the following two adjustments:

- — make sure that the little toe stays down in contact with the floor;
- — roll the foot slightly to the outside so that the bone on the inside of each foot moves up and in.

This will bring the opposite side of that bone down towards the floor making an 'even and equal' placement of the bones under the ankle knobs.

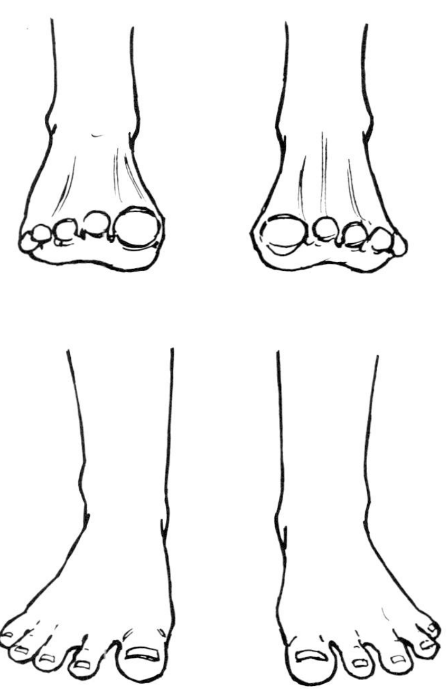

Do not overdo this movement or you will finish with your ankle twisted to the outside, which is incorrect.

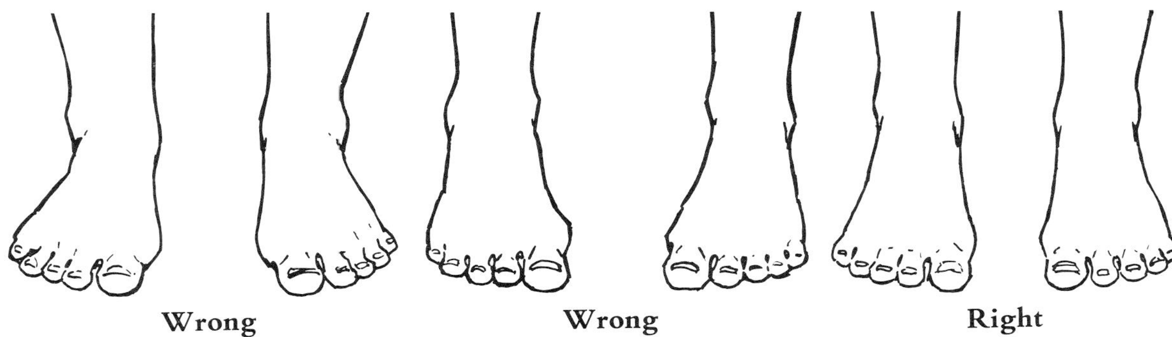

The outside edges of your feet should now be in contact with the floor, your weight should be off the joints of your big toes, and your arches should have lifted automatically.

If you have difficulty getting your big toes pointing straight forward and your feet are not parallel, you may, without changing the position of your toes, move your heels just about a quarter of an inch outwards, away from each other. Make sure you don't overdo this or you will end up with your toes pointing inwards. After you have practised the little toe will stretch more easily to the outside, the weight will be taken off the big toe, and you won't have to make this adjustment.

When you have checked all these points, lift your head and look straight forward.

Knees over insteps

Without bending your knees, move them forward so that the centre of your knee-cap is almost over your instep and you can feel your toes move well down into the floor. Do not lift your heels as you do this. This positioning creates your centre of balance.

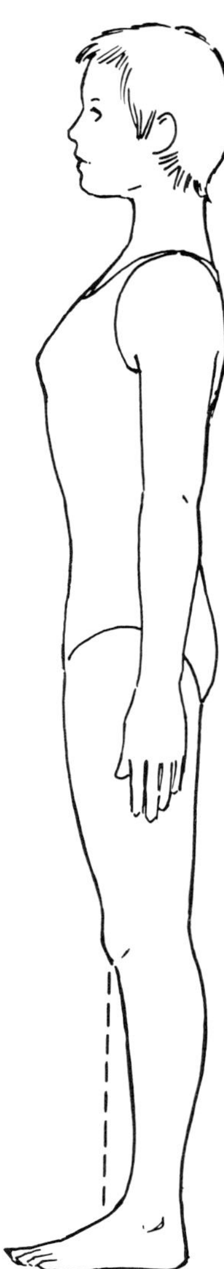

Tighten your knee joints slightly but do not lock them back hard. If they feel locked, lessen the tightening in the knees and move them over the insteps again.

You must constantly check that your knee-caps are in line over your insteps. Executing and maintaining the alignment depends on this.

Hip rotation

As you have already learned, relaxing the cheeks of the buttocks and directing the knees inwards affects the hip movement. We have done this several times as part of the Touch Knowledge. It is achieved in the same way when you are standing.

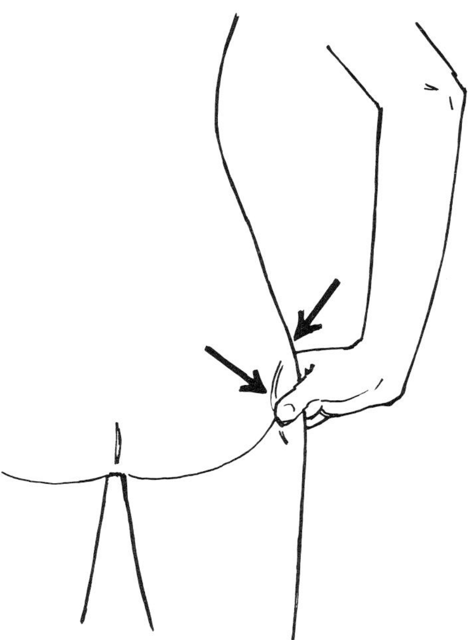

Place your hands low on your hip joints, thumbs behind in the depression where the sciatic nerve lives. Now relax the cheeks of your buttocks, increase the distance between your calves slightly and direct your knees inwards.

Remember that directing the knees inwards does not mean

pushing the knees together, it means having the knees directed slightly towards an imaginary central point between and in front of them. With your hands on your hip joints as you do this, you should be able to feel a slight rotation of your hips and some tightening in the front of your pelvis.

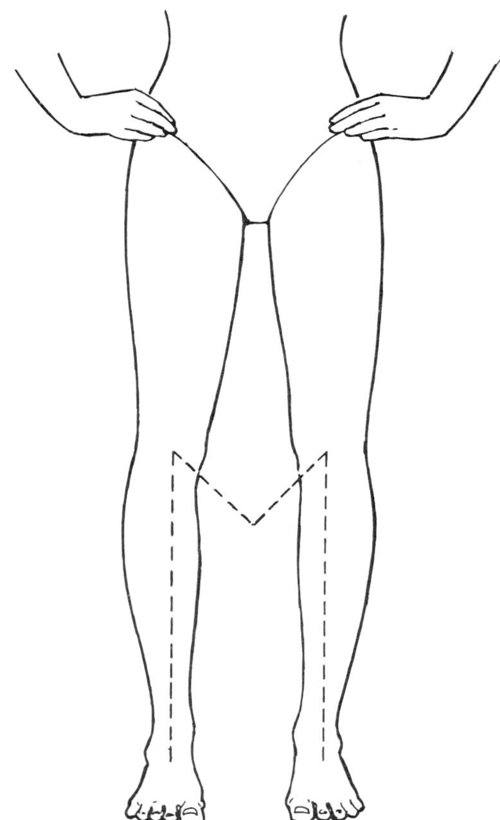

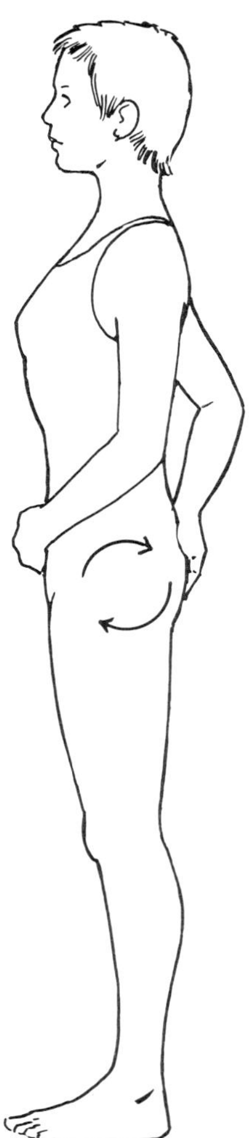

The pelvis adjustment

Place your left hand on your lower abdomen between your hip joints, and the palm of your right hand on your lower back with your middle finger on your coccyx. Push the coccyx down hard with the middle finger of your right hand as you firmly lift your lower abdomen up and into the front of the pelvis with your other hand.

Do not tilt your pelvis forward. It should have an 'even and equal' placement underneath your rib-cage. The position of the feet, knees and hips works to form a cradle for the organs within the pelvis. Supporting the abdominal organs in this way flattens the abdomen and at the same time helps to correct the curve in the lower back. The tightening into the front of the pelvis is essential in stretching the torso correctly. Also this low abdominal area is the important power centre for concentration of movement. It is the 'holds you together' place.

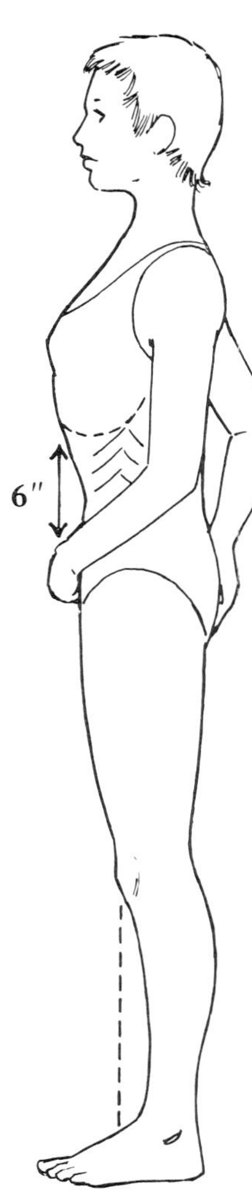

The spine

With your hands in the same position – holding your abdomen up and in and your coccyx down – start stretching your spine upwards from the coccyx.

Direct your attention to each vertebra in turn as you did during the Touch Knowledge. This will help you with a mental image of how to achieve this stretch.

As the spine stretches, the muscles between the upper and lower torso also stretch. Try not to push your rib-cage forward but help the stretch by lifting your rib-cage upwards. This is when your waistline should begin to reappear.

Since those 'in-between' muscles have probably shortened because of a curved back, there may be a tendency to go back to the stomach-out-hollow-back position. You counteract this by checking that

— your feet are straight and parallel;
— your knees are brought forward over your insteps;
— your hips are rotated so that your stomach is tightened

up and in, and your coccyx is down;
— you are not leaning backwards with the upper part of the torso.

All these adjustments help to maintain a positioning in what we shall call the pelvic cradle, the area into which you have moved the abdominal muscles up and in. These muscles held up in this area are the source of strength for the stretching of the torso and the straightening of the spine.

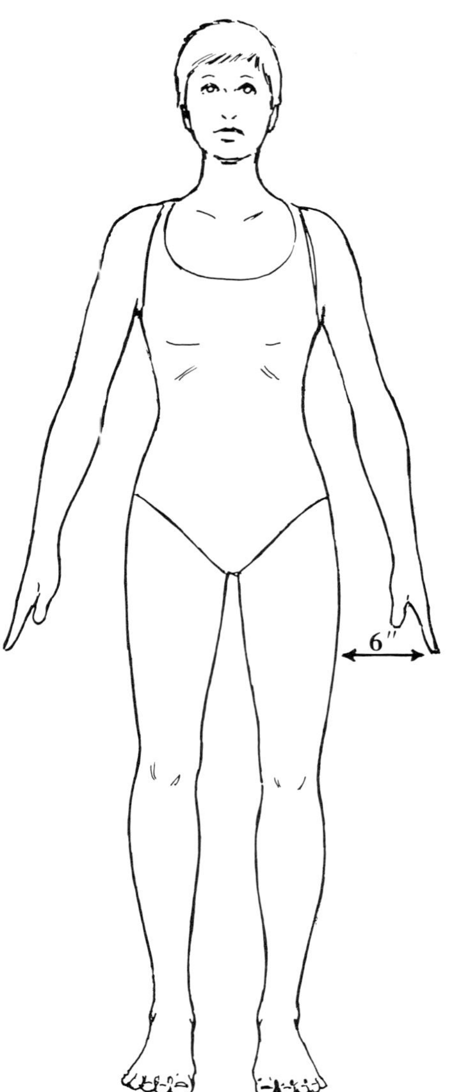

The shoulder rotation

When you have straightened your spine and stretched the 'in-between' muscles as far as you can without straining, remove your hands from your pelvis and put your arms straight at your side with palms facing inwards about six inches away from your thighs, all fingers held together.

Now do the same Shoulder Rotation as you did when sitting down for the Touch Knowledge: move your shoulders half an inch up towards your ear-lobes, slowly move them back just half an inch towards your spine, then lower them one inch straight down towards your elbows. Do not throw your shoulders back in an exaggerated movement, and make sure that you do not arch your back as you bring your shoulders down.

Check, when you finish the rotation, that you have not brought your shoulders right back to where they were when you started.

Straighten your arms completely: the elbows, wrists and the joints of all the fingers. This straightening from shoulder to fingertips is important. (Make sure you do not let your hands angle inwards from the wrist.) It helps to maintain the correct position of the shoulders and upper torso. It also keeps the muscles between the elbows and the ends of the fingers stretched sufficiently to counteract any tightening of the joints and clawing of the fingers.

Now, keeping your shoulders in their 'down position' and your arms straight alongside your torso, raise the centre of the breastbone upwards.

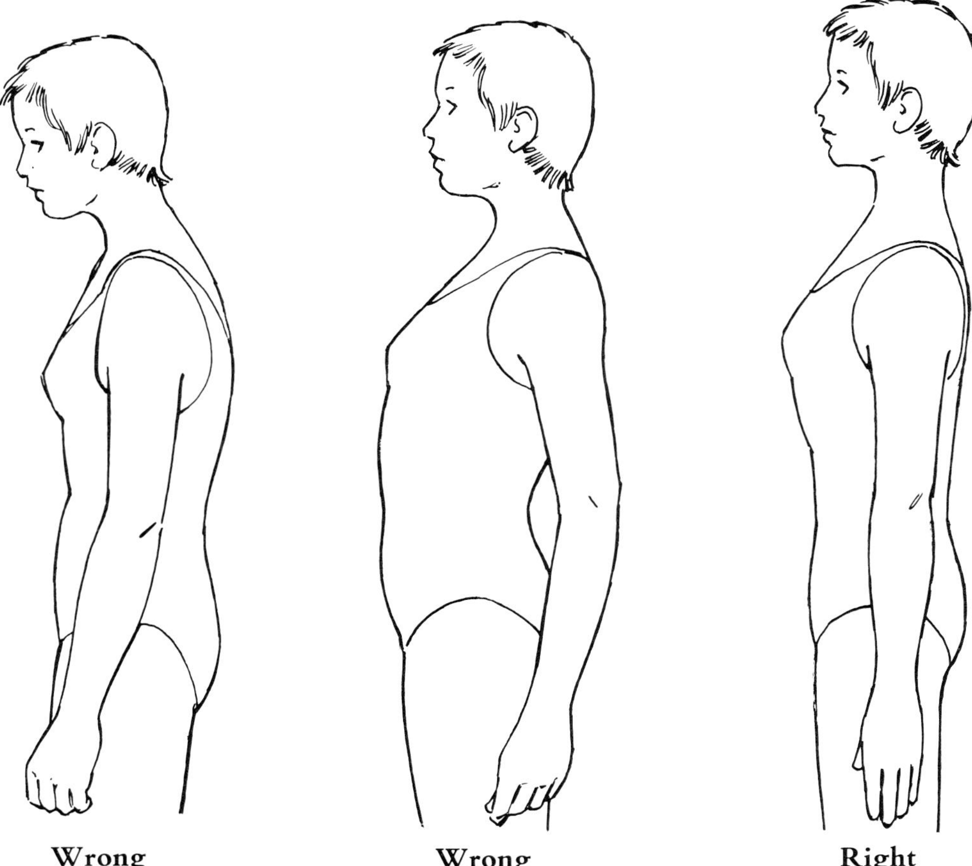

Wrong Wrong Right

The head and neck

With your eyes level and your chin at a right angle to your neck (not lifted or lowered), move the crown of your head well back in line with your spine. This creates a straight, crown-of-head-to-coccyx line.

With your shoulders lowered and your arms straightened, your breastbone lifted and your head back in line, the hinge of your jaw will tighten, moving the muscles of your face up and back.

Mentally check each of the movements executed without changing your eye position.

Hold this re-structured position for one minute only at the beginning. This position can create a new and unfamiliar sensation for your body, and, with so much going on, please don't forget to breathe!

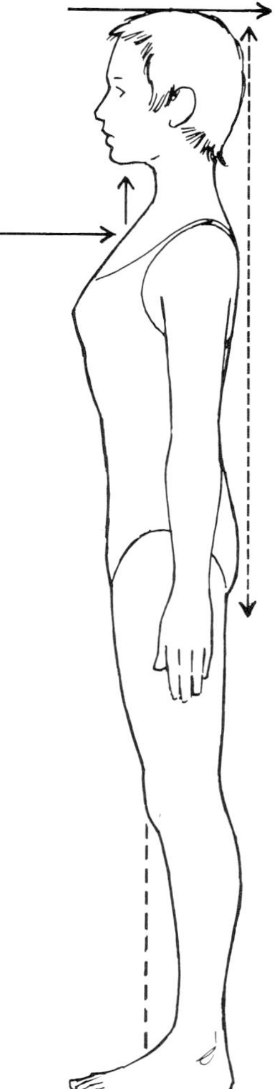

THE RELEASE

After completing the re-structured position, do each movement of this Release slowly without disturbing your alignment. Before you start, check that your feet are still parallel. Now clench your fists. Flex your elbows and bring your fists up in front of and level with your shoulders, palms facing inwards.

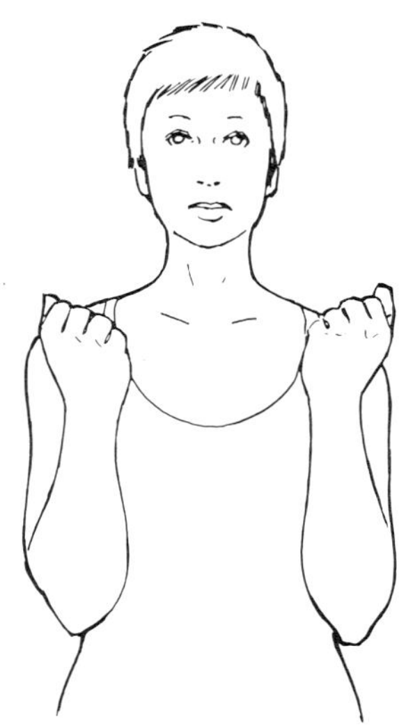

Take a deep breath as you raise your rib-cage and really tighten the lower abdominal muscles. Make sure that you do not raise your shoulders or curve your back as you do this.

The following movements should be done simultaneously:

1. Exhale as you flex your knees down about six inches in line with and over the insteps.
2. At the same time, bring the elbows forward (still flexed) to rest on the tops of the knee-caps.

Now lower your forehead on to the flat part of your fists, between the first and second knuckles. Check that

— your toes are spread so that the little toe is down, the big toes are facing forward and the rest of the toes are flattened on the floor;
— your knees are directly in line over the insteps, otherwise your ankles will roll;
— your abdominal muscles are pulled in tight and up as high as possible;
— your coccyx is brought down;
— your shoulders are kept down;
— the weight of your head is kept forward.

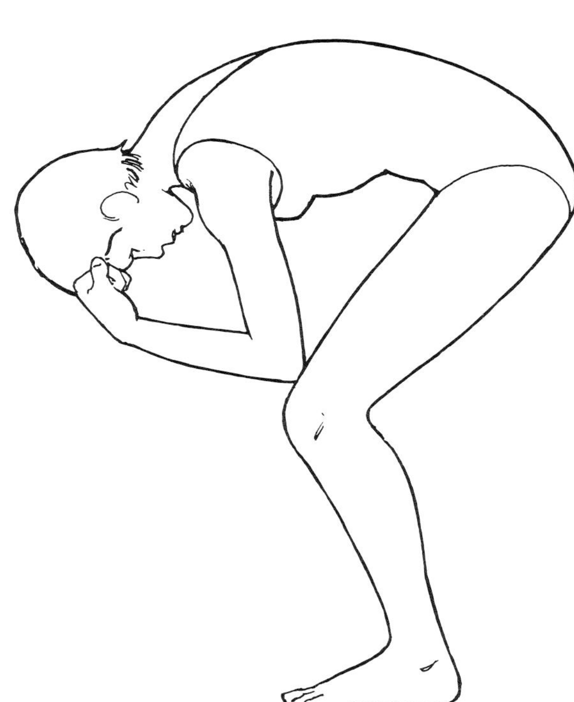

Now rock gently backwards and forwards in this position, alternately lifting the toes and the heels. Do this for about one minute, breathing naturally. This rocking is so soothing I have given you a time limit in case you go into raptures! When you are ready to come out of the release, make sure that you keep your coccyx down as you uncurl into an erect, standing alignment.

Lift your head, straighten your knees and back, and bring your arms to the sides of the torso. Check that your head is back in its correctly aligned position. You are now ready to do the Stretch.

THE STRETCH

Throughout this Stretch maintain your re-structured alignment. Turn your palms to face forwards and, keeping your arms straight, raise them to shoulder height. As you do the Stretch check that

— your shoulders stay well down;
— your arms and hands stay absolutely straight from shoulder to fingertips (this means straightening all the joints: elbows, wrists *and* fingers);
— your head is not dropped forward or tilted backwards but maintains its crown-of-head-to-coccyx line; your chin is at a right angle to your neck;
— you do not hollow your back.

Take a deep breath and clench your fists. Now, all at the same time:

— lift your toes
— spread your fingers
— open your mouth wide
— push out your breath with a loud, explosive A-A-A-H-H-H-H-H-H-H-H. . . .

This explosion takes all that energy you have created and brings it right out into the open. No 'implosion' here: everything is externalized and stress-releasing.

Once you have done these three exercises, the most difficult part is over. We shall use the same rules for everything else in the book.

Now walk around a little, using your new alignment as much as possible. You may feel a bit tin-soldierish but this disappears with practice.

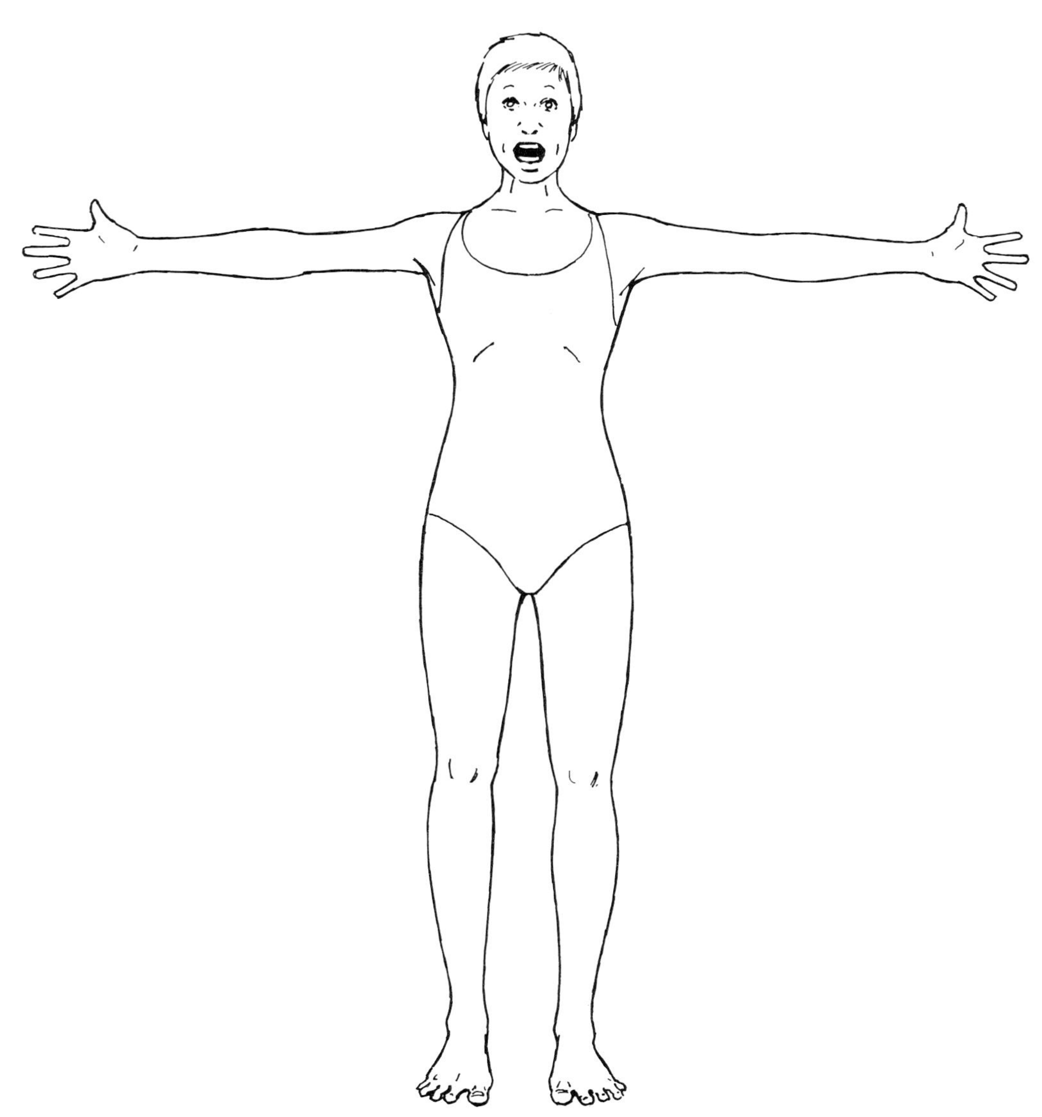

A-A-A-H-H-H-H-H-H-H-H!

Also, please note that, when your head is in line, the corners of your mouth go up more easily. It is easier to smile!

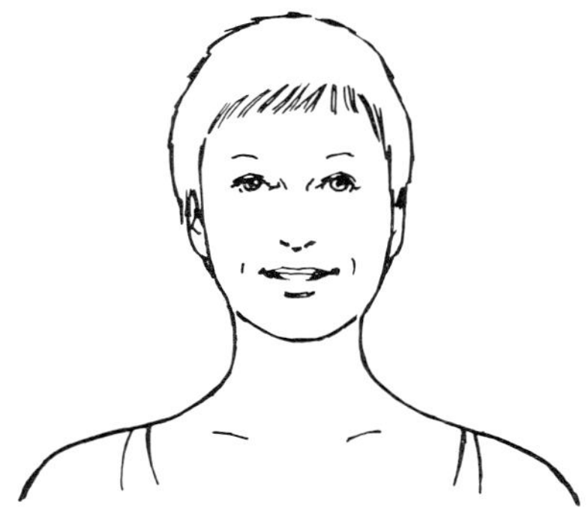

AFTER THE STANDING 3-SET

Once you've done this initial alignment, it will take no time before you start, almost unconsciously, to bring it into your daily living. In fact, after the first go at it you'll probably walk out of your room and immediately think of correcting everyone in sight. Please refrain, for all the obvious reasons. What I should like you to do is think about it. Let the knowledge *sink in* and, if you find yourself beginning to move the body as you think, that's fine. Take two or three days before going on to the Sitting Alignment.

However many days you take, try to do the Standing 3-Set twice on each of those days (or at least once), but do not go on to the Sitting 3-Set until you feel familiar and relatively at ease with the Standing. If a week is necessary, fine. However, barring major interference, I should prefer not more than ten days to pass.

THE SITTING 3-SET

I am now going to teach you the Sitting Alignment, with its Release and Stretch, in two positions. They will vary only because one will be done on the floor and the other sitting on a chair. Try the floor-sitting first unless physically you absolutely cannot – then go on to the chair. If you wish, and you have the time, you may do them both at one session. If not, run them as close together as possible – preferably the next day. In any event, read before you do.

SITTING ON THE FLOOR

Do you remember how you sat on the floor against a wall in the Touch Knowledge? That is how I should like you to sit now. In fact, much of that chapter is directly applicable here.

Stretch your legs out in front of you so that your feet are parallel and about six to ten inches apart. (The outer sides of your feet should line up with the outer sides of your hips.) Reach behind the cheeks of your buttocks and find the 'sitting bones'. Pull them back one at a time towards the wall. Then, with your hands still on your buttocks, spread the cheeks by rocking from side to side. These movements will simultaneously bring the upper thighs deeper into the hip joints and pull the lower part of the torso under and in line with the upper part of the torso. This brings the abdomen into a position where the muscles can be tightened, and the spine into a position where it can be straightened.

Be sure you feel both your 'sitting bones' in contact with the floor. This helps to stop the body from listing to one side or the other and the spine from twisting.

About this time those of you with shortened hamstrings along the backs of your legs are being given notice of their existence. You may flex your knees upwards a little to relieve the strain. But, if possible, your legs should remain straight.

In either case, flex your ankles, leave your heels on the floor and point your toes to the ceiling, with your feet still parallel and six to ten inches apart. Do not 'drop' the little toe down to the side but make sure all the toes are in a line straight across and facing the torso. Span your hip joints with your hands, thumbs behind, as you did in the Standing Alignment. Now direct your knees slightly inwards.

As you do this you should feel under your fingers a slight tightening of muscle into the front of the pelvis.

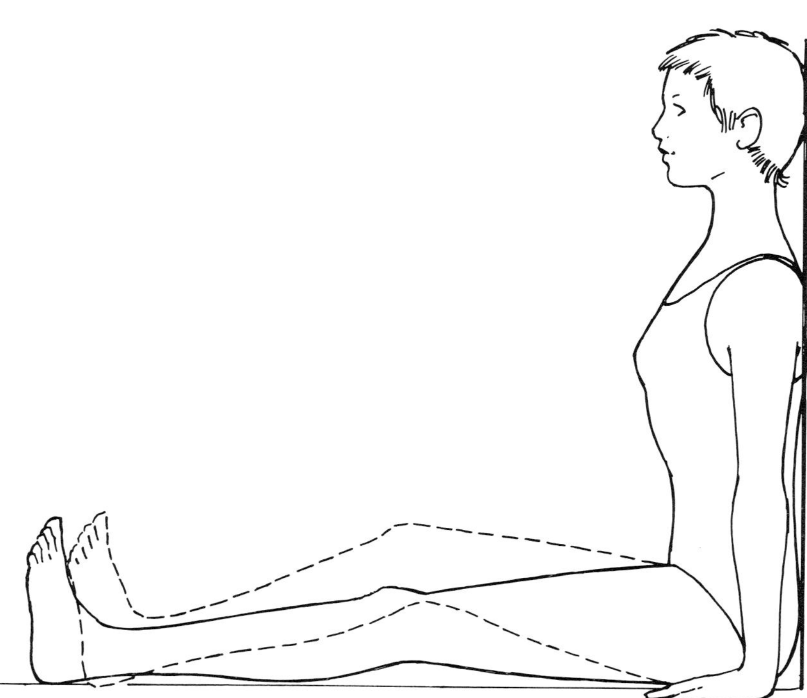

The arms and hands

Place your hands flat on the floor alongside your hip joints, palms down, fingers together and pointing forward. If your arms are long, you may have to move your hands *marginally* forward of the hip joints. In any case, do not angle your elbows outwards as that will bring your shoulders forward.

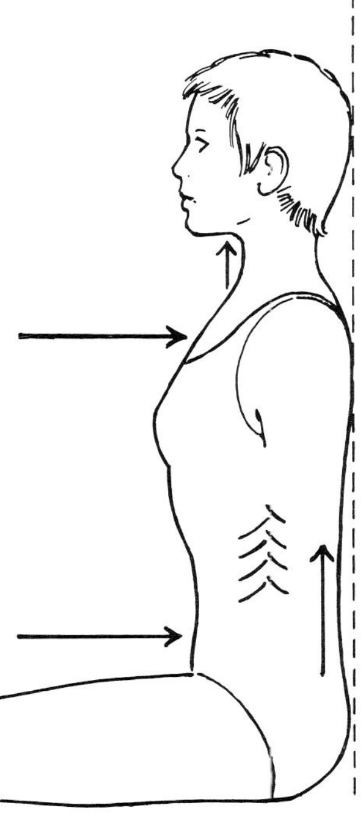

The back stretch

Bring the lower part of your back – three or four inches up from the coccyx – into direct contact with the wall, and do not let hell or high water move it away throughout the ensuing sitting instruction.

Now, mentally and physically stretch your spinal column and the muscles between the upper and lower parts of your torso upwards, by concentrating on each vertebra in turn and *moving it against the wall*. This movement duplicates the Standing Stretch, where the emphasis of pull is concentrated on tightening the lower abdomen ('cradle' or 'pelvis power') rather than arching the lower back. The stretch that is created by extending your toes upwards and moving your hips back permits the centre of the pelvis to tighten sufficiently to support the stretching of the spine upwards. This will also tighten all the muscles from the feet to the pelvis.

Don't forget to breathe!

When you have stretched three-quarters of your vertebrae against the wall, rotate your shoulders in the now familiar way – up half an inch, back half an inch, down one inch. Keep your elbows at the sides of your torso.

Now raise your breastbone (an inhale helps this), and stretch the tendons of your neck.

Move your head backwards. Do not raise or lower your chin while doing this, but keep it at a right angle with your neck. Your eyes should look straight forward. In your mind, see a long crown-of-head-to-coccyx image of your back along the wall. Breathe evenly, and hold this position for one minute only. Then immediately move into

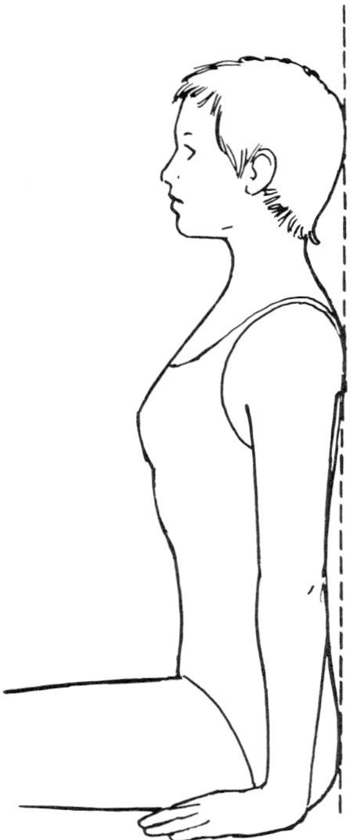

THE RELEASE

Push away from the wall and sit so that your knees are flexed and your feet are placed flat on the floor, parallel and the usual distance apart. Clasp your hands around your knee-caps, with your elbows flexed. Now straighten the elbows and, as the torso tilts back, make sure that the spine (crown-of-head-to-coccyx-line) is kept as straight as possible. Both feet should remain firmly in their positions on the floor. Really tighten the lower abdominal muscles. Keep tightening as you curve your entire spine forward, sliding your hands along the shin line. Come to rest with your hands clasped and your head on or between your knee-caps, or as close to them as possible. Relax your neck.

Breathe evenly for one or two minutes.

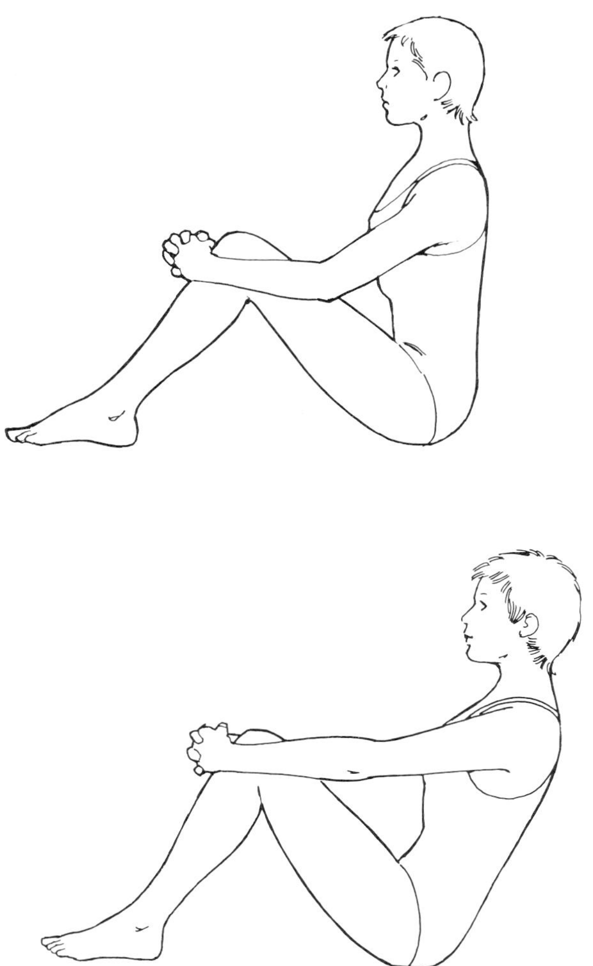

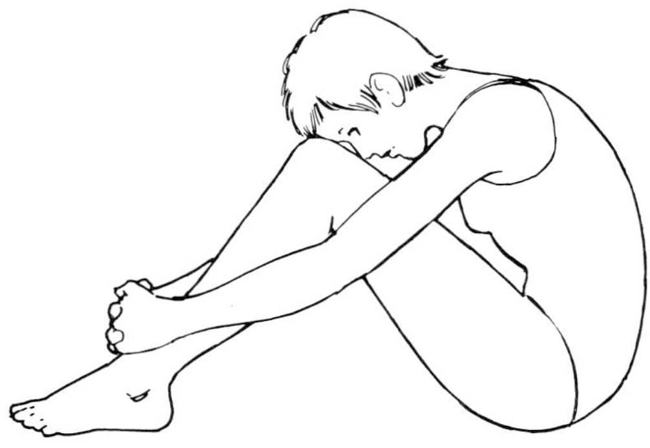

THE STRETCH

Lift your head as you straighten your back. Unclasp your hands. Open your arms with your palms forward. Straighten your elbows and lower your arms until you can place the tips of your middle fingers in line with the hip joints. Now, with your arms still straight and your palms still facing forward, raise your arms to shoulder height as you straighten your legs. Put your feet in their parallel position, toes pointing upward, and tighten the lower abdomen.

Without wasting any time, make a tight fist, take an inhale and all at once

— open and stretch your fingers
— open and stretch your toes
— open and stretch your mouth
— push out your breath with a loud explosive A-A-A-H-H-H-H-H-H-H-H. . . .

Quickly bring your knees to your chest and clasp them as close to your body as possible. This will help give support to your back, which has been without any for a few minutes.

When you are ready, get up, walk around the room, and register the new sensations in your body.

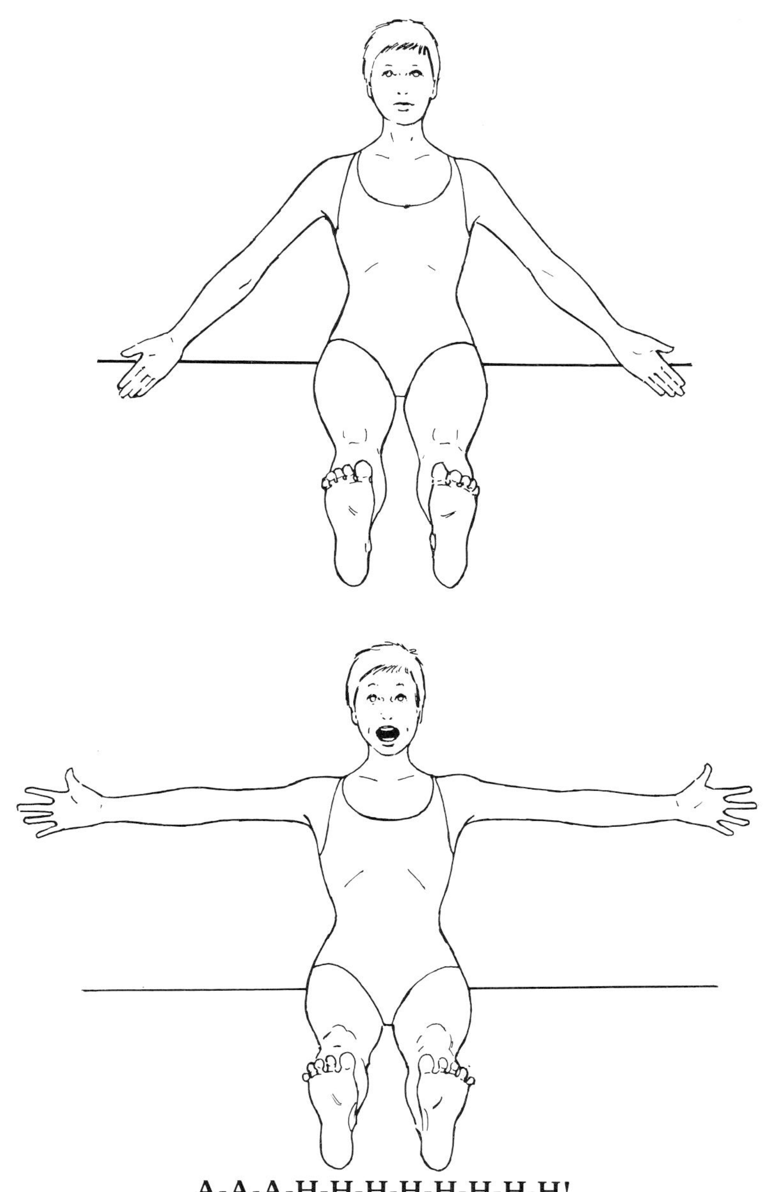
A-A-A-H-H-H-H-H-H-H-H!

SITTING IN A CHAIR

This is a great deal easier than the floor-sitting, and designed to be done more easily under everyday conditions. Remember that you are doing this as a re-structuring exercise. It is most certainly not a position in which you would normally place yourself (i.e. sitting on the edge of the chair). However, the basic principles apply whenever or however you sit in a chair. We shall discuss that later in Section II.

Place the chair in such a position that you can sit on it and extend your arms upward to shoulder height.

Sit down, and move your buttocks forward until the 'sitting bones' are on the very edge of the chair. Rock from side to side to spread them. Place your feet so that they are parallel and the outside of the foot is in line with the outside line of the hip. (Keep your feet the usual distance apart.)

Your knees, ankles and feet should form right angles, like this:

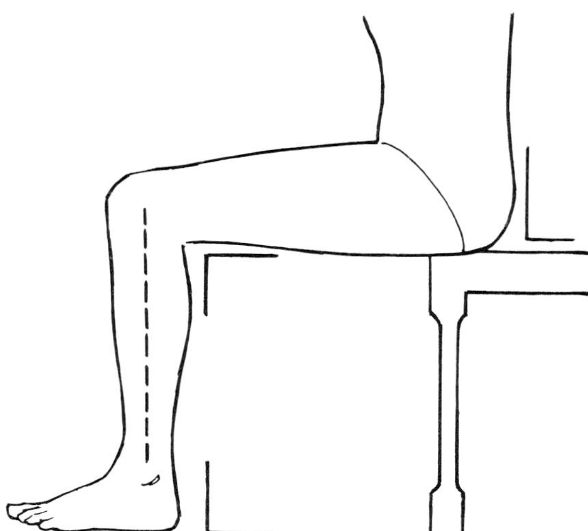

In other words, the ankle should be directly under and in a straight line with the knee.

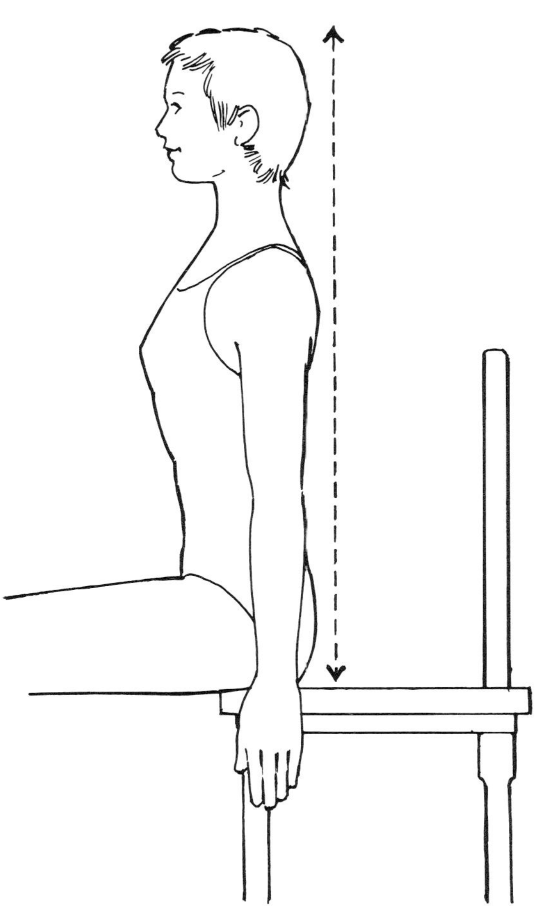

Lift your toes upward, spread them and place them down flat – the big toe straight forward and the little toe stretched to the side – just as you did in the Standing Alignment.

Direct the knees slightly inwards. Tighten the abdominal muscles up and in and at the same time move the coccyx down towards the seat of the chair. You may use your hands to effect this if you wish. Now start the spinal stretch exactly as you did in the Standing Alignment. Make sure you do not loosen the tightening into the front of the pelvis, otherwise your abdomen will drop forward and your back will arch.

Three-quarters of the way up remove your hands and let your arms hang down alongside your hips on the outside of the chair. Do the shoulder rotation, and then really straighten your arms from shoulders to fingertips. Make sure the finger joints are straight and you can feel a muscle pull right to the fingertips.

Stretch your neck back so your head is in line (remember – chin at a right angle), eyes straight forward and corners of the mouth lifted. Breathe, and hold for about a minute.

THE RELEASE

Make fists. Flex your elbows and bring up your fists so they are in line with and facing your shoulder joints. Tighten the abdominal muscles as you bring your elbows forward to rest on the tops of your knees. Place your forehead on the flat part of the fist, between the first and second knuckles, relax your neck, and keep your shoulders down. Now lift, first your toes, and then your heels, about six times. Stop, hold, breathe, and get ready to stretch.

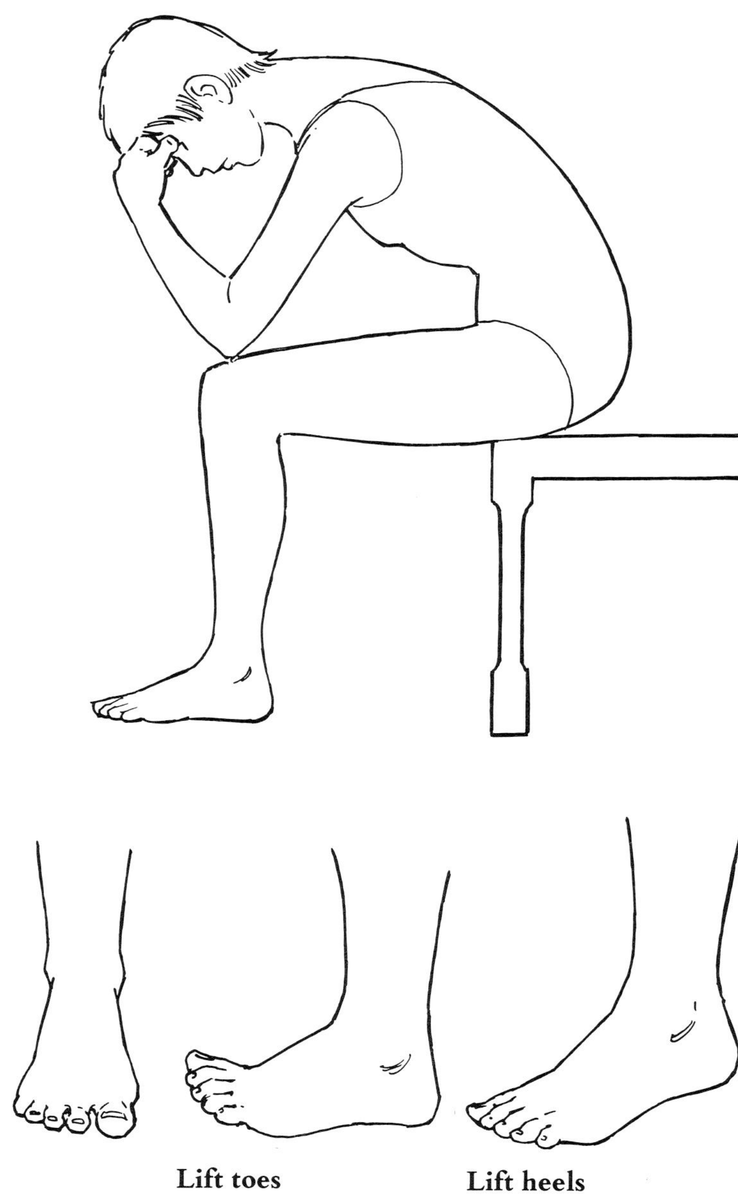
Lift toes
Lift heels

THE STRETCH

Lift your head and bring your hands, palms forward, to the sides of the chair, straighten your back and move your head back into crown-of-the-head-to-coccyx line. Tighten into the front of the pelvis – feel the 'sitting bones' on the chair and bring your coccyx down in line with them. Keeping your shoulders down, raise your arms, palms forward, to shoulder height.

Make fists.

Take a big inhale and all at once
— lift your toes
— open your fingers
— open your mouth
— and A-A-A-H-H-H-H-H-H-H-H. . . .

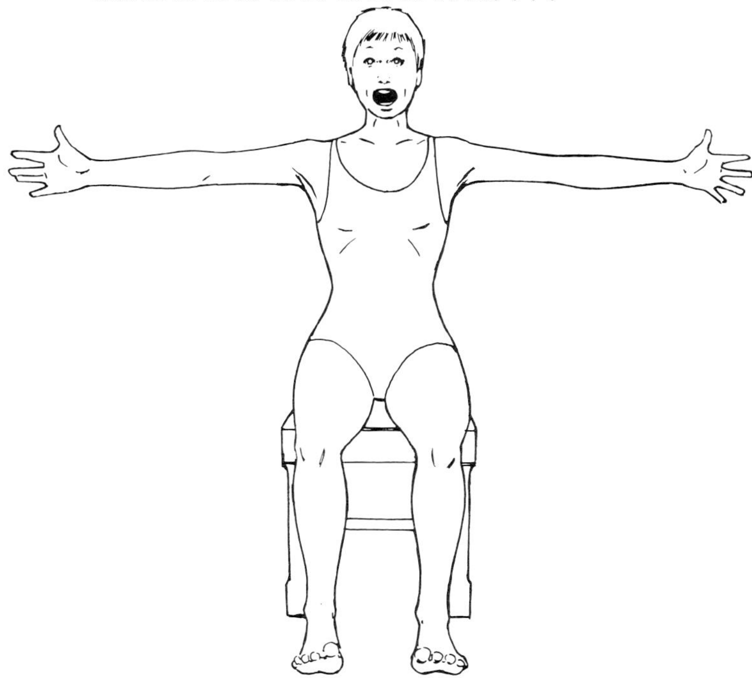

Get up, walk around the room – in fact, walk *out* of the room!

AFTER THE SITTING ALIGNMENT

Take three or four days to do the Standing and Sitting Alignment each once a day before you go on to the Lying Alignment. The floor-sitting will help stretch the hamstrings, so try not to neglect it completely. Also, think about the alignments from time to time. Using your own voice to tell you how to do it will help enormously.

When you have given yourself sufficient time, and are satisfied that you are ready to proceed further. . . .

THE LYING 3-SET

You are now ready to face (lying down) the third position. By now you must have got clearly in your head – and fairly clearly in your body – what all this is about. In fact, you might very well be able to do this one without my help, but for both our sakes let's not risk it. There are always a few specifics when you are learning that have to be made very clear.

If you want something to lie on, you may use a large towel, but personally I just lie on the floor.

Make certain you have enough room for the Stretch. That means room to extend your arms on the floor all the way up to shoulder height.

Be sure to read the instructions through first. For this position, particularly, it is advisable to use a tape recorder to put my words in your voice.

ALIGNMENT

Lie on your back with your legs stretched out, and your feet the usual six to ten inches apart. Flex your ankles so your heels are on the floor and your toes are pointing directly upward.

(Make sure the outside of the foot is brought up evenly with the inside: that little toe again!) With your hands, spread the cheeks of your buttocks (do not lift them up, just spread them horizontally from side to side) enough to move the coccyx down and to feel the lower part of your back come into contact with the floor. This will take the curve out of the lower back. If you feel you cannot maintain this contact with your knees straight, flex them upwards, but keep your feet the same distance apart and pointing upward. Try not to let your feet angle outwards, as they will be inclined to do. Your arms should lie straight alongside and about six inches away from your torso. Your palms should be facing the floor, your fingers stretched straight and held together. Throughout, the most important thing is not to let your lower back curve away from the floor.

Now tighten into the front part of the pelvis by directing your knees slightly inwards. Keep this pelvic area as your centre of concentration, as always, and gradually, vertebra by vertebra, stretch the spinal column along the floor. Don't forget to breathe. Now lift your rib-cage, but try not to disturb your spine against the floor.

Next comes the shoulder rotation. Keep it small. Lift your shoulder joints towards your ear lobes half an inch, back to the floor half an inch and straight down flat along the floor one inch. This should put your shoulder-blade area flat against the floor. Do not arch your back as you do this.

Now really straighten your entire arm from shoulder to fingertips along the floor. Extend your fingers flat, together and straight, with the palms down.

Raise your breastbone towards the ceiling. As you stretch your neck, keeping your chin at a right angle with your neck, try not to raise your chin as you stretch. This duplicates, with the exception of the hand placement, the standing re-structured alignment.

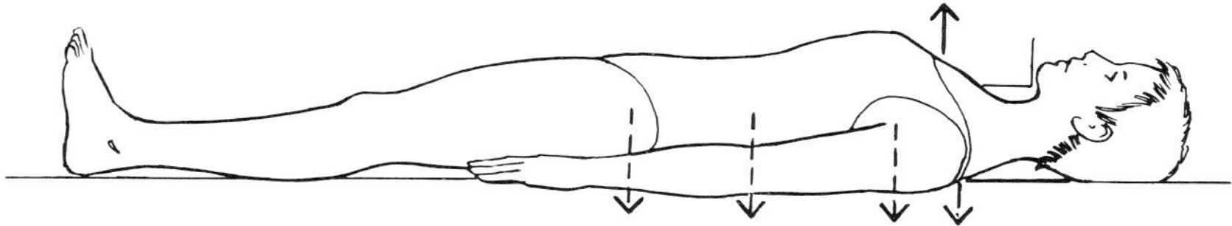

THE RELEASE

Keeping your toes pointing to the ceiling and dragging your heels along the floor, slowly flex your knees upwards as far as possible. While you do this, be sure those lower abdominal muscles stay tightened and the lower back stays flat on the floor (they do go together!). With your knees still flexed, lift your feet in the air, cross them at the ankles and clasp your arms around your legs – somewhere under the knee-caps. Bring your clasped legs towards your chest slightly – keep tightening on the abdominal muscles.

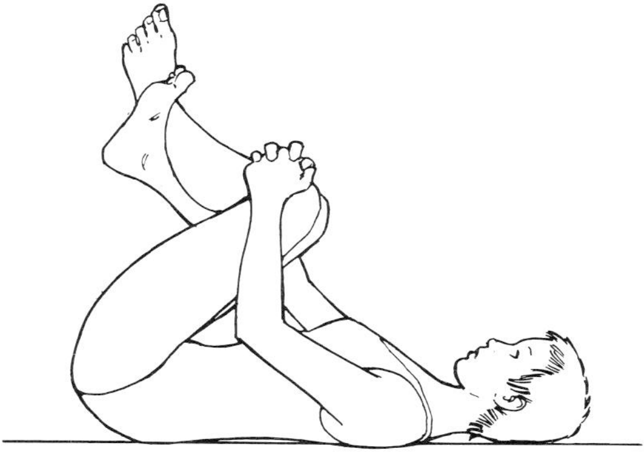

Release any tension in your neck by lowering your chin towards your chest.

This should feel delightful. If you like, while you are breathing away, you could let your feet, still crossed, move up and down in a small bouncing movement – this can be soothing and tranquillizing.

THE STRETCH

Unclasp your arms and place them at the sides of the torso, palms facing upwards. Uncross your feet and place them soles down on the floor, with your knees still flexed. (Do this fairly quickly so you do not arch your back.) As you straighten your knees, bring your arms straight up along the floor until they are in line with the shoulders (palms still upwards, shoulders down). At this point the knees should be straight, your ankles flexed and your toes pointing to the ceiling.

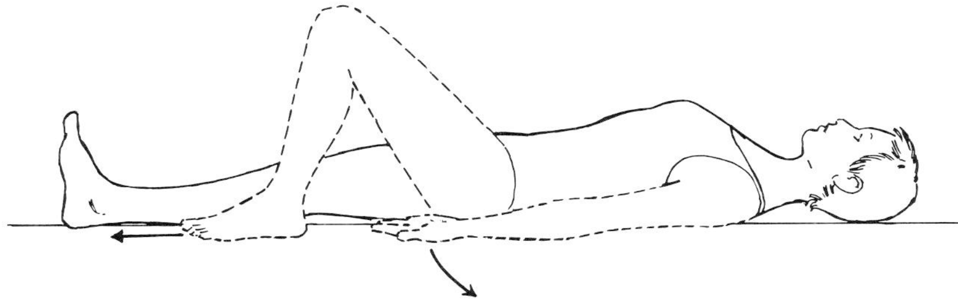

Once more, make a tight fist, take a big inhale and all at once

— open and stretch your fingers
— open and stretch your toes
— open and stretch your mouth

— push out your breath with a loud explosive A-A-A-H-H-H-H-H-H-H-H. . . .

Just lie there and enjoy! Only one more point: try not to let your feet relax outwards. This opens the pelvis and arches the back. Learn to relax with the feet, loosened, straight forward, or even turned in a little. Unnatural as it may seem at first, it is well worth the effort.

AFTER THE THREE 3-SETS

You are now ready to go public. You have learned and become familiar with the basic tenets of your exercise survival kit. These 3-Sets, coupled with the next two chapters in this section and using the fundamentals in your everyday activities (see Section II), put you in a wonderful position to – that's enough – simply put you in a wonderful position!

Now here is your schedule, so far, for getting it straight and keeping it straight:

One 3-Set three times every day (or almost)

The Standing 3-Set
Do this when you get up in the morning. Your body is cramped from sleep and you will actually be shorter. By re-aligning your body to your full height, you will face the day straighter and taller.

The Sitting 3-Set
Do this in the kitchen – in the office – wherever, and do not hesitate to do the release and stretch. If questions are asked, just say, 'A-A-A-H-H-H-H-H-H-H-H!'

Try to do the floor-sitting about three times a week. It is worth it for gradual stretching of the hamstrings.

The Lying 3-Set
Do this on the floor, or even in bed without a pillow. If in

bed, do try not to injure your bedfellow (if you have one) on the Stretch. This could cause resentment, and in severe cases the loss of a companion!

Try to fit these in, as recommended, as we go on to the next chapter.

THE TRIANGLES

These triangles will give you a simple, rapid mental check on your correct body alignment.

I am going to give you very specific headings in this chapter, and then equally specific instructions. By the time you have come back to this chapter from the previous instruction (and have been doing the Alignments on a daily basis) you should have the technique well in hand. You are now ready for more and here it comes! I am actually, finally, going to ask you to use the mirror. It would be wholly advisable to use one that reflects you full length, otherwise you may find yourself checking isolated parts. We have already established that you are a whole person, *and* a person of many parts, and we want to be able to see it all.

Question: What will the Triangles do?
Answer: You will learn to use the points and lines that make up the triangular areas as imaginary guide marks to check and improve the alignment. By mentally focusing on the Triangles and the parts of the aligned body they contain, you will be creating for yourself manageable areas. You will use the mirror as a visual check.

In addition, the Triangles can work and help correct or prevent a twisting of the spine to one side or the other. By looking in the mirror at certain lines the Triangles define, you will be able to observe whether one hip – and, it usually follows, one shoulder – is higher than the other. You will then learn how to make certain adjustments (nothing major, just simple ones such as shifting your weight) in order to correct this misalignment. For example, creating a straight line from one shoulder to the other and then a straight line across the hips results in two parallel lines. The spine can then be stretched straight between them.

When we get going you will see what I mean.

Question: How do I do the Triangles?
Answer: First read, record and follow the instructions along the way.

Stand up and face the mirror. Adjust it, if necessary, so you can see your entire body from toe to head.

Now go through the Standing Alignment (but do not do the Release and Stretch). Make sure, after making the final head adjustment, that you do not disturb it by thrusting your face forward to peer into the mirror. Your eyes should be looking directly ahead and your head back in its aligned position.

Without disturbing your head position, direct your eyes to find one horizontal line – the top of the window, the bottom line of a picture frame, the mirror top. Bring your eyes back to their straight-ahead position and use the horizontal line you have found to extend straight across your eyes.

The second line you create is parallel to that one and goes straight across an imaginary line underneath the point of your chin. The third line, also parallel to the first two, extends from one shoulder tip to the other across the collarbones. Opposite is an example of how they and you look if they are not parallel.

We are now ready to create the Triangles. Just remember that they are simply three imaginary lines that connect three points to form triangular areas around part of the aligned body.

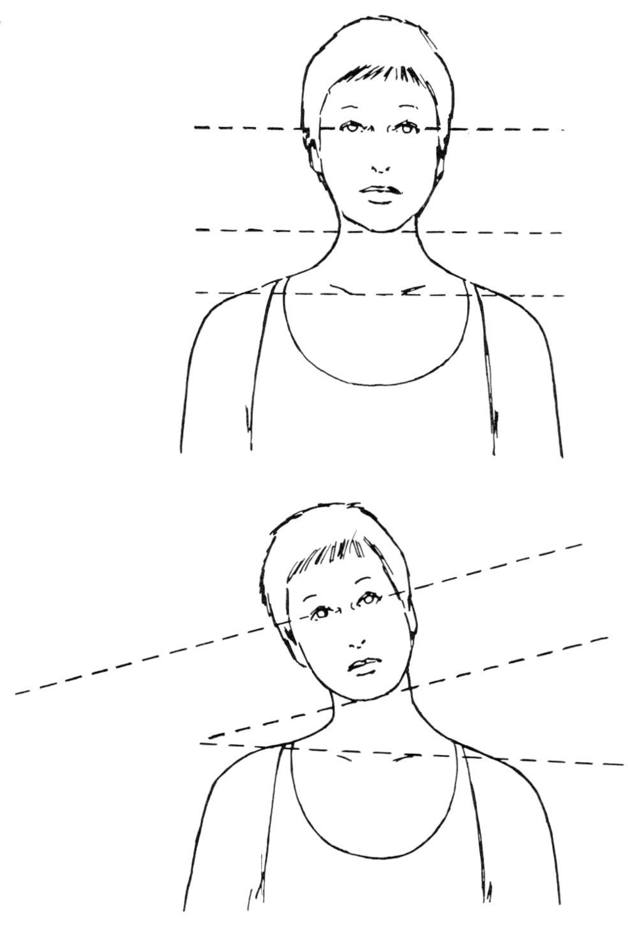

The first triangle

Imagine three points:

(A) is the crown of the head
(B) is the right shoulder
(C) is the left shoulder

In your mind, connect these three points with straight lines – and you have the head, neck and shoulders contained in a triangle.

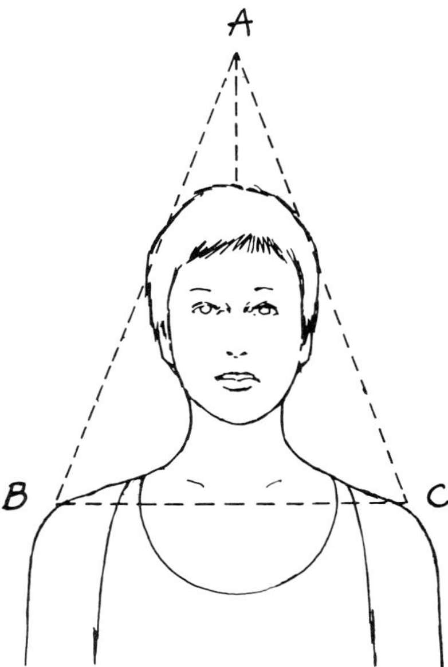

Use these points to remind you of the alignment precepts that

1. By keeping your head moved back to (A), it is kept in line.
2. By using (B) and (C) as points of reference, you keep your shoulders pulled down.
3. The straight line formed between (B) and (C) is, as you will learn, necessary to keep the spine from twisting.

The second triangle

This one is a partial overlay of the first that will extend straight down the arms of the fingertips.

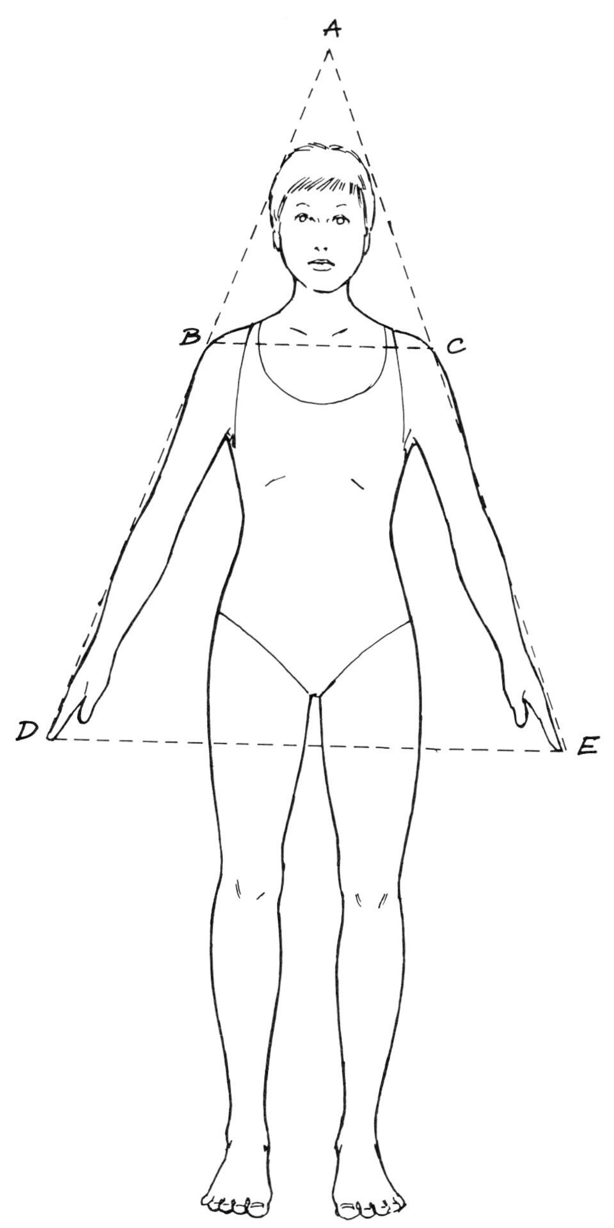
A
B
C
D
E

Here are the points to connect:

(A) the crown of the head
(D) the fingertips of the right hand
(E) the fingertips of the left hand

This Triangle connects the head and shoulder area to the arms and torso.

By stretching your arms and fingertips along the sides and into the points of the Triangle (B) to (D) and (C) to (E), you are aided both in raising the breastbone and in stretching the torso upwards. Both movements help to keep the head back in place.

The third triangle

This one will define the pelvic area. If you think of this triangle as inverted and following the lines of a bikini, front and back, you will be on the right track.

In this Triangle

(F) is the crotch
(G) is the right hip
(H) is the left hip

Connect these points, and you have the front part of a string bikini!

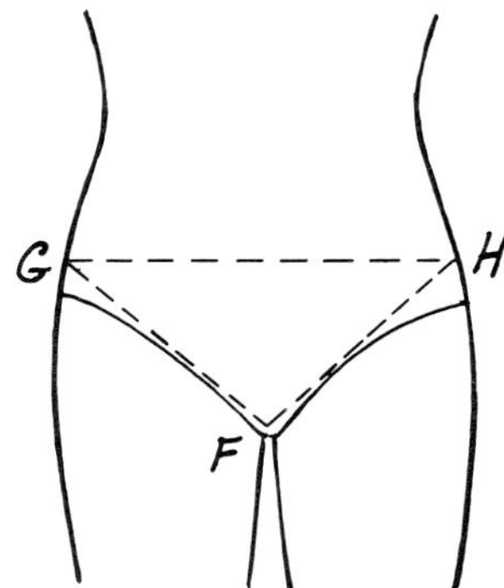

By defining the front sides of the bikini (F) to (H) and (F)

to (H) you are provided with specific lines to use for tightening into the front of the pelvis.

The straight line across from the hip points (G) to (H) should be parallel to the shoulder line (B) to (C) and is important for getting the torso laterally aligned and in correcting the spinal twist.

At the back

(I) is the coccyx
(J) is the right hip
(K) is the left hip

Connect these points and you have the second – and sometimes better – half of the bikini.

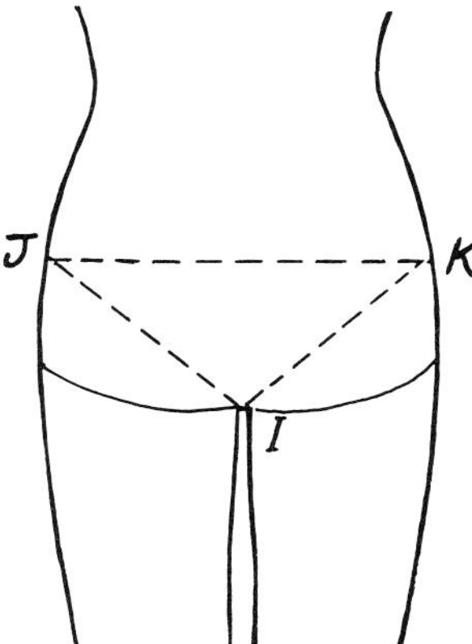

By using (I) as the placement point for the coccyx being 'brought down' (a case where not seeing is believing), you will be better able to envisage this adjustment. The line across from (J) to (K) will provide you with an awareness of where the flattening in the lower back should take place.

The fourth triangles

Back to the foundation! We shall work with both feet at the same time. You can see them in the mirror without disturbing your head position.

The points on each foot are:

(L) the centre of the ankle joint
(M) the joint of the big toe
(N) the joint of the little toe

Connect the points so that each triangle defines the front and top of the foot.

By using the stretch line across the toe joints (M) to (N) as a point of reference, you can see (M) as the big toe kept forward, and (N) as the little toe stretched to the side on the floor.

You can use the point (L) as the place where the 'even and equal' adjustment of the ankle joint is maintained.

These triangles, divided down the centre, provide a clear 'plumb line' reference for the central balance over the instep.

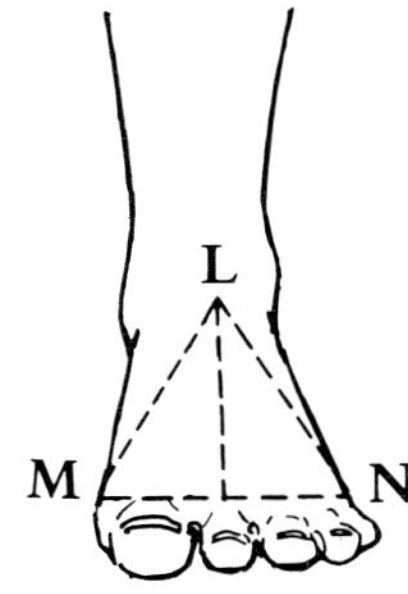

Finally, the mirror has its moment!

There you are all aligned, looking straight ahead and impressively arrayed in imaginary triangles. There is one more important correction that must be carefully investigated. So stop – please sit down and read the following.

Earlier on I referred to the twisting of the spine and how we could make certain adjustments in order to correct or prevent it. Now we are going to attack the problem.

First let us look at these two drawings.

The drawing on the left has the body weight divided equally over each foot. This permits the bottom hip line and the top shoulder line to be straight and parallel. Between these two the spine can then be stretched in a straight line from the coccyx to the crown of the head.

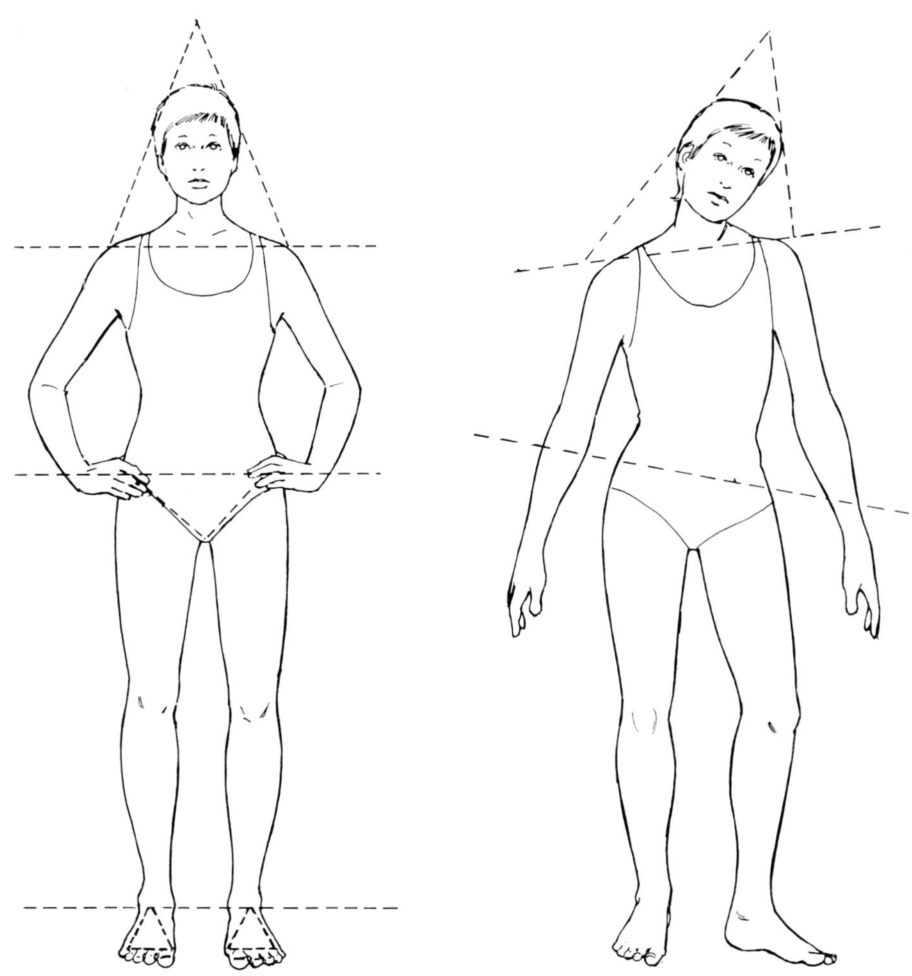

The drawing on the right has the body weight over and down on its left foot. This puts the top and bottom lines (still parallel) on a diagonal slant. Between these two the spine stretched upwards must, to some degree, be twisted.

So how can we correct it? First you must see and feel the correction. It would be a good idea to record the following instructions:

1. Stand up
2. Face the mirror
3. Align the body completely
4. Put in and 'see' the four triangles.

Now place your hands around your hip joints, thumbs behind, fingers in front, with the fingers of each hand pointing towards each other. Make sure you feel they are spanning the joints at the same place on each side.

Look carefully into the mirror.

Are the fingers of each hand absolutely opposite the other, or are they higher and lower?

Do you feel under your fingers a difference in the hip bones, one being higher than the other?

Does one knee look higher than the other?

Look: is one shoulder higher than the other and the head held to the side?

If you see or feel none of these differences, you are unique.

In most cases people are right-handed, and so the weight is usually over the left side with the right side brought up; so for simplicity's sake I am going to give the correction method for the majority. You simply reverse it if your left side is brought up.

Keep looking closely into the mirror.

Shift the weight slowly from the left side on to the right by pushing your hand down on the right hip (you should feel the movement under your fingers) until:

1. The fingertips of each hand look directly opposite each other.

2. Your hips 'feel' in the same places under your fingers.
3. Your weight feels and looks more over the right foot.

This movement should also have helped to raise the left shoulder and lower the right. If it has not done so sufficiently to create a horizontal line across, rotate the right shoulder and feel it pulled down until this is achieved. The head should now look quite straight.

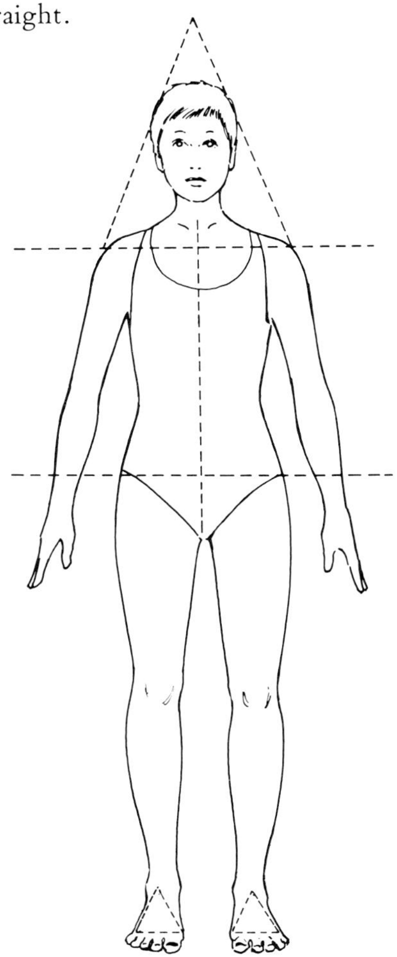

Now close your eyes and register how the effects feel on your feet – in your hips – in your spine – in your shoulders – in your neck. You cannot take the mirror with you but you can take the *feel*.

Now, how about opening your eyes and doing a Release and Stretch?

QUESTIONS AND ANSWERS

Question: How often should I do this in front of a mirror?
Answer: As often as you can, checking the effects until the 'feel' becomes really familiar.

Question: Can I really correct or prevent a twisted spine by doing this?
Answer: Just as you can improve and help to prevent vertical misalignment by knowing how to correct it, and bringing the corrections into your daily life, so can you with the lateral. The two alignments work to help each other.

Question: Is there anything else I can do that might be beneficial in correcting this 'twisting'?
Answer: One other thing – you can do this in the Alignment when you come to lifting your rib-cage. Place your hands on either side of the rib-cage. Feel (and look in the mirror to see) whether the one side is extended outwards more than the other. With your hands, using a 'typewriter carriage' motion, shift the extended side over until you can see and feel that the two sides are evenly placed in the centre of the torso.

Question: Are there any other positions in which I can do these Triangles and the lateral adjustments?
Answer: Of course – in the Sitting and Lying re-structured Alignments. Once learned, no contradictions – the technique is consistent.

KNEE FLEXES AND BOUNCES

To this point in the book, your instruction has focused on learning and maintaining the Alignments. Now we are going to start exploring the pleasures of using the Alignment in movement.

The aligned body will benefit more from all movement than a misaligned body. These energetic and continuous movements which we are going to learn will help to provide a balanced programme of exercises.

Be sure to read through first, and you may want to record.

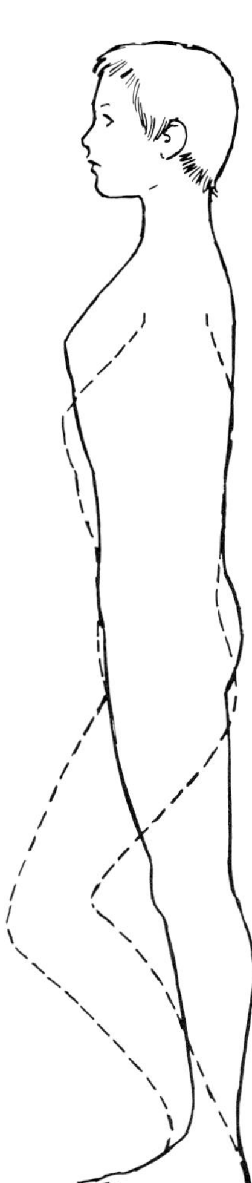

THE KNEE FLEXES

Question: What is a Knee Flex?
Answer: It is a flexing of the knees that results in a lowering of the aligned and vertical body. Throughout, the body remains vertical, and the alignment rules are consistent. The return of the body from this flex to its original position simply requires a reversal of the movement.

Question: How are they done?
Answer: 1. Align your body in the re-structured standing position.

2. Keeping everything in its aligned position, slowly flex your knees into an angled position just over and in line with the central lines of balance of your feet (to remind you of the last chapter, they are the dividing lines of the triangles). Stop this movement downwards when you feel a pull along your shin bones. Do keep both your heels and your toes on the floor, and your feet very much in their parallel six-inches-apart position. Try not to lean backwards or forwards.

In the drawing on the left the coccyx is lowered in a direct line downwards to a point between the heels, not too far; then you will feel that pull along the shin bones. If this doesn't register, it probably means your torso is collapsing downwards and dissipating the pull as you will see in the centre

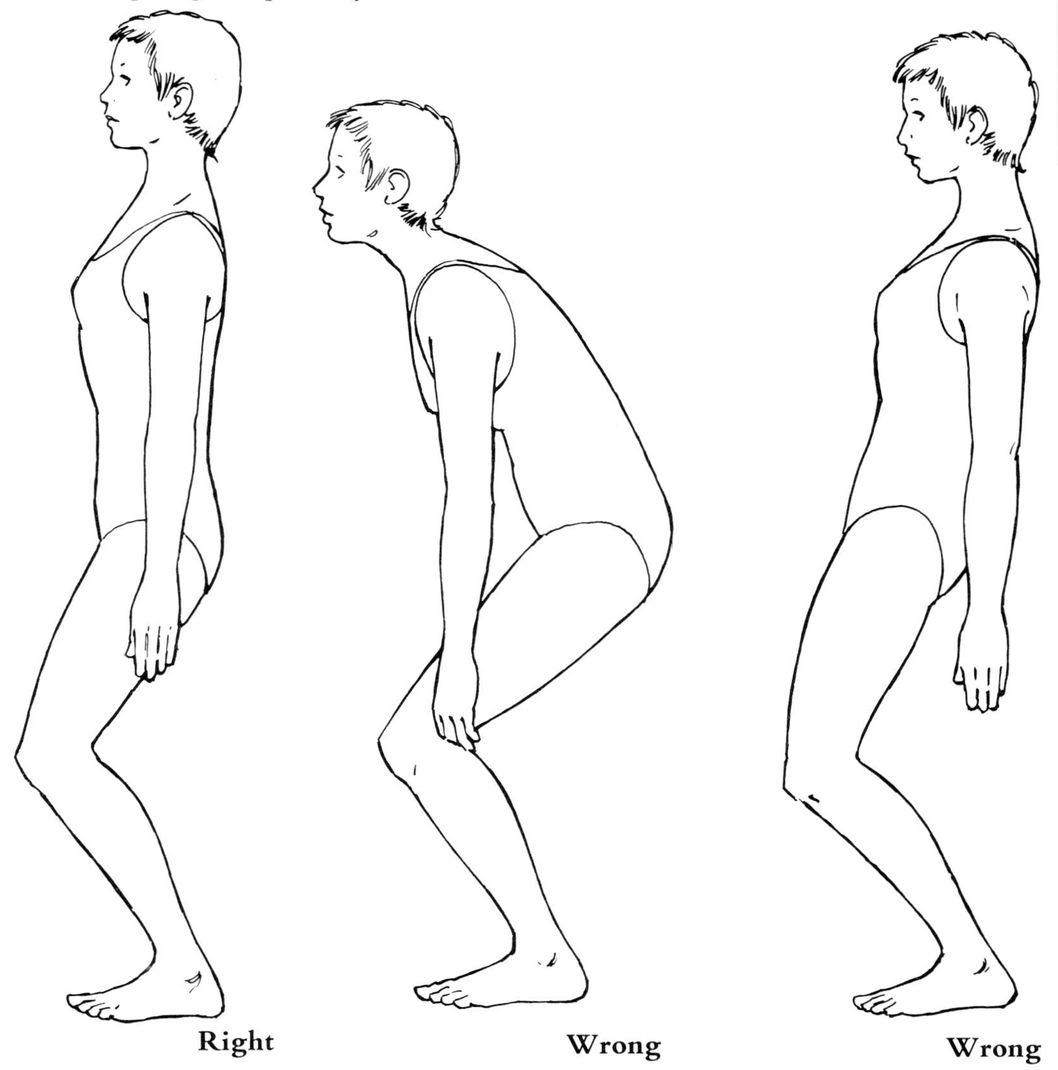

Right **Wrong** **Wrong**

drawing. In this position you will feel a 'curving in' in the waist and abdomen. Try lifting your rib-cage and lowering your shoulders. If you lean backwards, as in the drawing on the right, you will feel the upper thighs 'pulled'.

Hold the correct position for a few seconds.

THE RETURN

Slowly straighten your knees until you are back to the original standing position.

Take a few breaths and try the combination of Knee Flex and Return again. (Incidentally, if you can remember, it is a good idea to take an inhale before you start, and exhale as you flex your knees.)

Do several of these combinations, until they feel familiar, then do a Standing Release and Stretch. Take a breather and a walk around – sit down, and read on.

I am going to give you a plan of action for developing the 'feel' and the stamina for going on to the bounces.

In fact, to those of you who do not, for any reason, want to try the bounces, these knee flexes can work, in themselves, as energetic and continuous exercise.

A PLAN OF ACTION

You will want to develop the Knee Flexes gradually so that you never sacrifice the alignment for speed of action or length of endurance. When you find that is happening, STOP. Here is a suggested building programme before you start the bounces.

Take three slow counts to go down into a flex, then, at the same speed, three counts to come back up. Do four sets of these in succession and then, at the same speed, on the fifth – three counts down – hold three counts – three counts up.

Keep building on this pattern, using your ability to maintain the precision of the alignment as a guide to extending the number and the speed of sets you should do. As a rule you will find that the precision starts to slacken at the same time as the breath starts to quicken. Develop the number of flexes gradually, until you have got to the point where you can do about six sets of the above to a fairly rapid count. Then gradually go on to doing them without any 'hold' in the knee-flex position.

This will take you days to develop, and for some of you even longer. There are those, as I have said, who will want to continue building on this knee-flex pattern and never take to the air. But for those of you who will here is a sensible test before you embark.

Do twenty Knee Flexes straight through without a rest to a fairly fast count. When you can maintain the Alignment and be just a bit short of breath, you are ready for take-off.

THE BOUNCES

In these Bounces, it is the vertical line of the body, cushioned by the flexed knees, that prevents the jolts and helps to develop the bouncing momentum. (Rather the same principle as the pogo stick.) Also, the lifted and expanded lung area the Alignment creates assists in getting in the extra oxygen needed. Maintaining the re-structure throughout is not only important – it is essential.

It is probably a good idea to record these instructions.

1. Align the body in the Standing re-structured position.
   - *a) Look down. Check that your feet and ankles are absolutely correctly aligned and six to eight inches apart.
   - *b) Look up. Bring your head back into its aligned position with your eyes directed straight ahead.
   - *c) Make sure your spine is very straight, coccyx down, abdomen tightened.

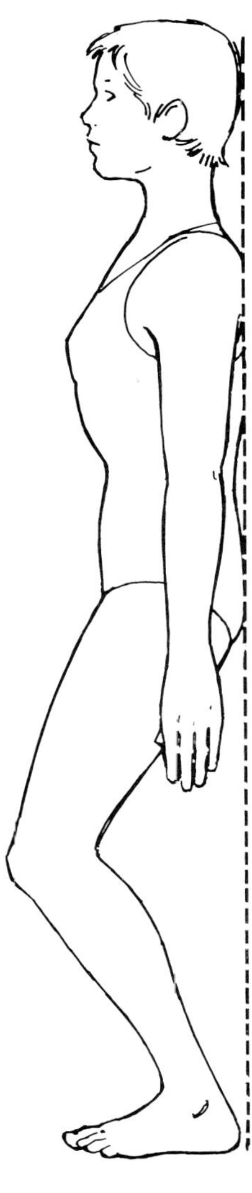

*d) Check that your shoulders are brought down, and your arms are very straight through to the fingertips. (*These are points you can keep reminding yourself of throughout.)

2. Do a Knee Flex and STAY in that position.
3. In your mind, create an extension from the crown of the head going straight to the ceiling, and another from the coccyx going straight to the floor between the heels. Think of that line as a vertical 'string' that will help to keep you in line as you bounce up and down.
4. With a small springing action bring the entire body off the floor without disturbing ANY PART of its Knee Flex position.
5. Return both feet to the ground aligned and at the same time (one count) still in the Knee Flex position.

In the air your feet should have remained parallel to each other and pretty much parallel to the floor, so that when you land they will be in the right position to bounce against. Do not land and bounce on the balls of your feet. This is a very common tendency. Another is one we shall tackle right now. Take a look at your feet after you have bounced once. See if the old faults have made themselves evident. Are your ankles pushed in and the feet angled out? If they are, you will be bouncing on your arches and weakening your ankles. Correct these faults if necessary. Now look up and re-align the body. This time, because one is really more difficult to do than a number, we will try three in succession.

Take a few breaths before you start – Knee Flex – then with a continuous, rhythmic count, keeping the Bounces small, with no pause in between,

GO
1-2-3-STOP

Good!

Check your feet – correct them – look up. Think of the vertical string helping you to bounce.

A few breaths – and

GO

1-2-3-STOP

Great!

Now return to the Standing Alignment – Release – Stretch – walk around a little – then sit down for a rest, a read, and a review.

Before we go to the developing your bouncing programme, I have a few suggestions on how to improve the quality.

If you are thudding heavily, instead of bouncing lightly, don't blame it on your total body weight – eight-stone wonders can thud just as readily. There are probably two reasons why this is happening. The first is that misalignment in the body creates a situation where the various parts cannot assume responsibility for their own weight. In other words, in misalignment one part pushes down on another. This collapse makes you heavy on your feet. In order to lighten the burden, you align. If you are 'thudding', you are probably collapsing on your landing.

The other reason can be the height of the Bounces. Until you are quite proficient keep them small and continuous – and, of course, knees flexed throughout.

One more suggestion that will improve the quality and enlarge the benefits: keep the corner of your mouth lifted. You certainly do not want sagging jowls being bounced!

Developing a programme of bouncing relies very much on the same tenets as the Knee Flex programme. Maintaining the Alignment is the key to success. (Incidentally, warming up with Knee Flexes before you do any Bounces is a splendid idea.)

Throughout, you must feel and listen to what is happening to you. If you do six Bounces and you feel that is enough, *stop*. Then try to hold yourself in that position (knees flexed) for six counts and *feel* if you are ready to do six more. Listen. If your breath is coming very fast, wait another six counts, then assess the situation. You can either do a *Return* and *stop*, or do a few Knee Flexes (Knee Flexes are Bounces in a minor key), or more Bounces.

Finally, you should be doing Bounces (or Bounces combined with rapid Knee Flexes) continuously.

The prime rule is to develop the Knee Flexes or Bounces in increasing numbers slowly over a period of time. Doing them once or twice a day is ideal – even three or four times a week is acceptable – but the business of doing very energetic exercise in fits and starts is simply asking for problems. However, as we shall see in Section II – 'Living It Straight' – everything we do in daily life that constitutes continuous motion, such as walking or going up and down stairs, done in a way that uses the body correctly, can supplement all rapid-movement programmes.

Before you go on to Section II, give a thought to your individual needs. Do you *need* to go through Section I again? Do it. Would you like to get used to your 3-Set routine for a bit longer? Fine. Listen to your needs and feel what is right, and then you will be ready to start applying your new knowledge to your everyday life.

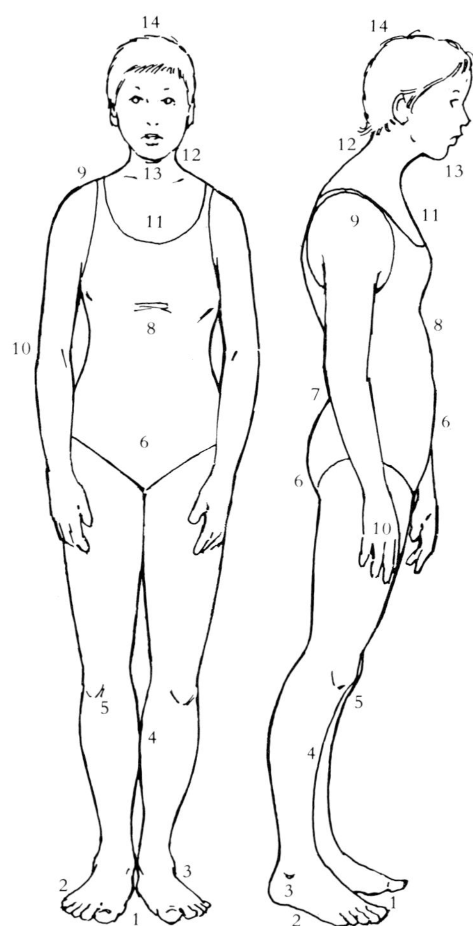

Incorrect

1. Feet and toes angled outwards
2. Outsides of feet not in full contact with the floor
3. Ankles pushed inwards
4. Calves pushed inwards towards each other
5. Knees 'sagged' and directed outwards
6. Buttocks clenched, abdominal muscles loosened and dropped
7. Lower spine curved
8. Upper part of torso slumped down onto lower, thickening the waist
9. Shoulders slumped forward
10. Joints slightly bent from shoulders to fingertips
11. Breast-bone lowered
12. Head dropped forward, curving upper part of spine and neck
13. Chin dropped
14. Head-to-coccyx line curved

STANDING ALIGNMENT

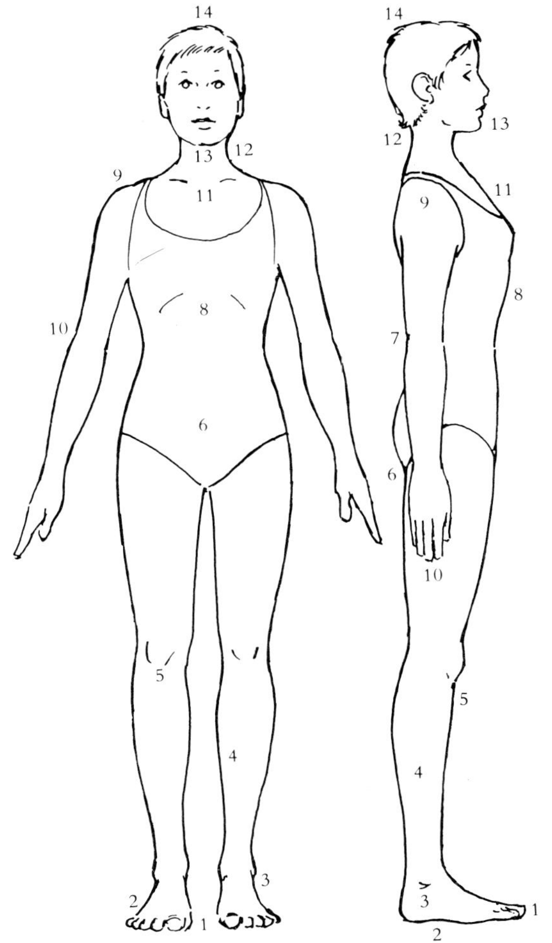

Correct

1. Feet parallel, toes straight forward
2. Outsides of feet positioned to have full contact with the floor
3. Ankles 'even and equal' under ankle bones
4. Calves opened slightly outwards
5. Knees 'lifted', brought forward over the insteps and directed slightly inwards
6. Buttocks relaxed, coccyx brought down, abdominal muscles tightened upwards and inwards
7. Spine straightened upwards
8. Rib cage lifted, stretching the muscles between the upper and lower part of the torso, narrowing the waist
9. Shoulders rotated down
10. Joints straight from shoulders to fingertips
11. Breast-bone raised
12. Head brought back, straightening upper part of spine and neck
13. Chin level
14. Head-to-coccyx line straight

LIVING IT STRAIGHT

At one point in my teaching there was a particularly good-looking, physically impressive young man who came regularly to my follow-up classes. In the first part of these classes I always give a one-to-one personal check-up: How is it going? How does it feel? etc. He was always more than enthusiastic, alluding in a modest way, with a shy, almost self-deprecatory smile, to his work, its demands from the public and the benefits of having an aware, aligned body in his profession. All very provocative stuff, in view of his good looks. Speculation ran wild. I do not think a consensus ever emerged as to what he actually did, but opinion leaned heavily in favour of something 'artistic'. Some, however, had far more esoteric convictions. Finally, curiosity won, and at one class, when he had just made his usual declaration of love and appreciation, the lady next to him said, 'What do you do for a living?' He turned his ever-so-aligned head to look at her, gave his shy smile and said, 'I sell life insurance.'

From this you will begin to see that 'living it straight' can prove beneficial in the most unlikely situations. The principles of the Alignment that you have mastered can be applied to every part of your life, not just the times that you mentally allocate to 'exercise', and in this section I will give you some tips on how to use the Alignment in all your daily activities.

By now, you have seen and felt the positive effects of doing the 3-Sets on a regular basis. You must be aware that you *look* a great deal better now that you are straighter – and *feel* better. So why not protect your investment? That is what this section is about. It will provide suggestions that will make the positive effects you already feel work in a continuing and self-feeding cycle. Every movement that you make, in the right position, becomes positive exercise, and the more you do, the easier and more natural it will become.

Let's take one simple example: standing. There is no such thing as *just* standing. In the first place, there are all those involuntary muscles working away all the time. In a corrected position your entire body – every part that functions – benefits from the correct position. But if you are standing in an incorrect position you are creating pressures that have an adverse effect on the functioning of your internal organs. For example, have you ever thought how little space is left for your heart and lungs to function when your shoulders are hunched forwards, or what happens to the digestive organs when you stand so that your stomach is pushed out in front of you? Just as standing becomes corrective exercise when you are in an aligned position, even nodding or shaking your head is a movement for improvement or detriment, depending on your body position; all simple daily activities done correctly reinforce your strength and your ability to maintain the Alignment, and the positive results will increase accordingly.

If you continue to use yourself correctly, your muscles become strong enough to begin to 'voice' their training. For instance, when you feel the strains and pressure of driving a car, your developed alignment muscles will tell you to ease down your shoulders, get your back straighter and place your feet in line over the pedals.

It is logical that joints positioned correctly function better, remain stronger and are more flexible, because they are being used in a way that conforms to their basic design. This results in better blood circulation. Take the same joints and position them so that they are working against their basic design and they will suffer, and the circulation too will suffer. One universally accepted opinion is that good blood circulation is a major factor in preventing and relieving rheumatic and arthritic aches and pains. Sitting down in an aligned position in a chair not only prevents back strain but also exercises the ankles, knees, hips and shoulder joints correctly. These and many other benefits will become clear as we proceed through the examples in this section.

I shall try to provide a fair selection of activities, and suggest how to integrate the Alignment into them. However, if your life-style is more idiosyncratic, I am sure you will be able to make some creative adaptations yourself. So let's go on to living it straight, starting with a modified basic standing position. This version, called the Mini-Alignment, not only looks good but travels well, and can be done inconspicuously before even a close audience.

THE MINI-ALIGNMENT

Question: What is a mini-alignment?
Answer: A mini-alignment is what you can do when you want to maintain the basic principles of the full alignment, but modified just enough so that the effects in appearance and feel are more relaxed. Since by now you have practised and 'own' the full alignment, you may find that your body has begun to assume the mini-alignment position by itself.

Question: When do I do it?
Answer: It is designed for everyday use. You use it on a daily basis as you are using yourself: standing, sitting or lying. It is a 'one count down' version that will help to keep you from going back to the old habits – and the old pains. Remember, however, that it is in addition to the 3-Sets, not instead of them. The 3-Sets are your 'musts' – the Mini-Alignments are your 'as often as possibles'.

Question: How do I do it?
Answer: Start by doing the Alignment as quickly and expediently as possible. Use the key words in your head, and keep the movements small and subtle.

Here are the key words of the Mini-Alignment. Carry it out in this order.

— FEET (straight forward, ankles adjusted)
— KNEES (directed slightly inwards, knee-caps lifted)

— HIPS (rotated, coccyx down, front of abdomen tightened)
— BACK (straight and stretched)
— SHOULDERS (rotated and down position, breastbone raised)
— ELBOWS (alongside torso)
— HEAD (back in line with the spine)

When you have finished the adjustments, take a larger inhale and, on the exhale, still maintaining the general re-structured line, let the entire body relax down about one inch. As a result you should see and feel the body moving into a still aligned but relaxed position, not into a misaligned and slumped position.

THE MINI-STRETCH

Here is an on-the-spot Mini-Stretch that can be done whenever you feel the need of an instant let-out, physically or emotionally.

You are in your aligned, or mini-aligned, position (standing, sitting or lying). Take a deeper inhale and at the same time make tight fists and close your eyes. On the exhale, open your mouth, push out the air, stretch your fingers and stretch your toes.

Even if you have shoes on you can still stretch the muscles of the feet, but try to make occasions when you can do the Alignment and Stretch without them.

WALKING

Walking is your best, most available, and probably most functional form of movement or exercise.

Even if you omit the Bounces, give up Knee Flexes, sell your tennis racket and throw out your running shoes, you will be fine if you take a good walk.

Question: What is a good walk?
Answer: A good walk is one that is done with your feet moving one after the other in their straight-forward, ankles-adjusted, position. (Remember, the American Indian was famous for his stealth and speed moving in this manner.) Your knees should be kept in line with your ankles as you extend your legs in a long straight line from your hip joints. (Do not raise the legs too high or you will goose-step!) On each step you let the heel come in contact with the ground first, then get the toe line down as a push-off for the next step. The coccyx stays down and the centre of the pelvis acts as your concentration power-point for the lifting and straightening of the torso. Your shoulders are rotated down, and your arms hang and swing along the sides of your torso. Your head should be back, in line so that you are not leading with your chin. Your breastbone should be held quite high, and you should *move*. Hold your spine stretched and straight and extend your legs from the hips. Your torso line should not be broken either by a caving-in at the waistline or by a sway or curve in the lower back.

Steps moving from hips become strides.

Get the image? Think movement, and MOVE.

If you are carrying shopping bags while walking, try to hold them so they are extensions of the lines from the shoulders to fingertips, along the sides of the torso. If your shoulders are slumped forward, these additional weights will make you bend out of shape.

Another help is to divide the weight you are carrying into two shopping bags evenly distributed on each side – balancing the burden.

If you are carrying a weight in front of you – a box, a bag, or, more importantly, a baby – keep your shoulders down and your elbows as close as possible to the torso so that you are supporting whatever you are carrying from underneath – a bit like shelf brackets.

Habitually using a shoulder-strap bag on the same side is not a good idea. Try to switch sides periodically. I know it will feel strange, but strangeness often opens up new forms of awareness.

Good walking needs some practice in imagining the move-

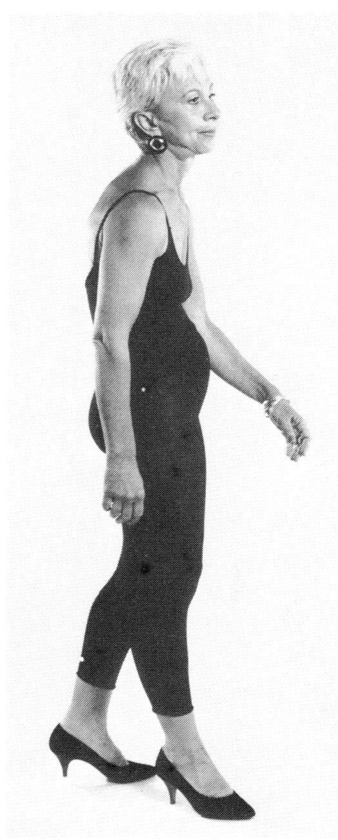

Wrong

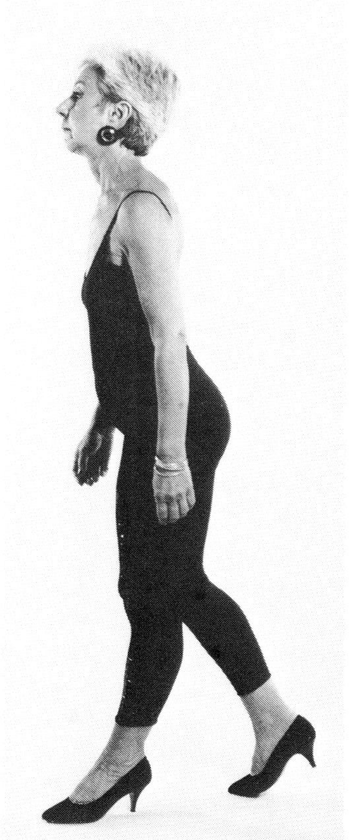

Wrong

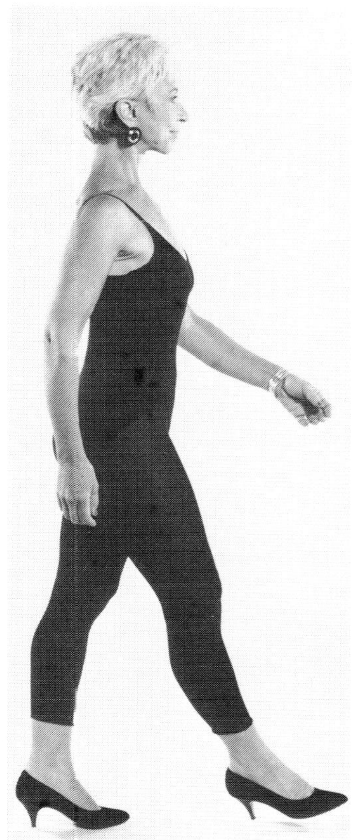

Right

ment before you do it – but not very much, because by now you own every one of the raw ingredients.

1. The body aligned means each part can assume responsibility for its own weight.
2. Each part assuming its own weight responsibility means the weight will not be collapsed down on to the feet.
3. Because the weight is not collapsed down on to the feet you will feel lighter and move more easily.
4. Feeling lighter and moving more easily should give you pleasure, and you will look better.

THE FEET AND SHOES

Question: What about shoes?
Answer: In my opinion, there is no way to deal with this question alone. I believe it is necessary to give consideration to feet and shoes, or feet in shoes, before any objective or helpful thinking on this matter can begin to take place. My own years in ballet provided an ideal situation for evaluating this subject, and undoubtedly my personal concern (have you ever seen a ballet dancer's feet?) acted as the catalyst. Were the *pointe* shoes the culprits – or was it the 'turned-out' technique – or both, or what? These questions were my initial concerns, and the answers provided the basis for what later emerged as my technique of body alignment.

In my experience, through years of looking at, and working with, literally thousands of pairs of feet (no two pairs alike), I have seen as many bunions, corns, flattened arches and weakened ankles in people who have worn 'sensible shoes' as I have in people who haven't.

There is a primary consideration, certainly not limited to the appendages we call feet, and that is heredity. It has been thoughtfully, accurately and impossibly stated that 'we should be wise in our choice of ancestors'. I cannot remember the number of times I have heard women in my classes say, 'I have feet just like my mother/father!' Yes, *father*, and I would not want you to think that this look-alike reference implied they were delighted with what had been passed on to them. On the contrary, they were almost always referring to classically bad feet, and I doubt if too many of their fathers had spent a great deal of time in shoes with three-inch heels.

So – we are born with idiosyncratic feet. Then, as infants, we crawl around on the ground and, at some point, usually at the urging of anxious (albeit good and loving) don't-let-our-baby-be-the-last-one-in-the-street-to-walk parents, we stagger to our feet in the best – and probably most desperate – way possible. Just to get up there requires us to push ourselves into any position to achieve the objective. The classic infant stagger is usually one where the feet are pushed out and flattened, the bottom stuck out behind, and the head charging well forward to try to balance this whole precarious manoeuvre – not unlike the look so common in elderly people who have never been taught how to correct the initial mistakes.

It has worked – we are up – but only in the way anything works when we must do *something*, but we really don't know how. We should be prepared to investigate a better way, if there is a better way of doing it.

Question: How does one learn to correct the causes of the misaligned stagger – and what does this have to do with shoes?

Answer: Out of shoes or in shoes, the feet come first. Walking barefoot will not correct the misaligned foot. It will, however, help you to use muscles in your feet, and once the position of the feet is corrected it can become an important exercise in itself.

Low-heeled shoes will not correct the misaligned foot, but they are probably more comfortable, and marginally less damaging, than high-heeled shoes. High heels will not make the corrections either, but can accentuate the faults by pushing the weight on to the front part of the feet.

Put any foot that is misaligned into any shoe and it is still the same foot in the same position, but encased. You then move the weight of a misaligned body down on to these feet and the original problems are enormously compounded.

There is, in my opinion, only one answer: you must learn to re-structure your feet and your body. You will then be able to wear shoes with your feet positioned correctly in them and your re-structured body will help to maintain this correction. Even high heels are manageable if you don't wear them for so long that you go back to the old habits of misalignment.

What about orthopaedic shoes? OK – but what happens when you take them off? Were stomach muscles ever strengthened by wearing a girdle? Like all things that prop you up, that is *all* they do. If you really need this, fine. But how much better if you can develop the means to do it on your own. Using the foot muscles in the correct position and without shoes on a regular basis is the best way to develop this support.

WALKING IN HIGH HEELS

As you can see in the pictures of me walking in moderately high heels, it is clearly a matter of very right and very wrong. Heels on shoes lift the body up from behind, and as this happens the torso will tilt forwards. To compensate for this, you should bring the coccyx down as much as is necessary to bring your torso back into its aligned position. As you walk you keep the coccyx down, and concentrate on tightening the muscles into the front of the pelvis to reinforce and strengthen this position. Try to walk from the hip line in front, and not from the lower back. Remember, if you are wearing high heels, all the instructions I have given you on walking apply, but to a much greater degree, in order to counteract the imbalance and maintain the alignment.

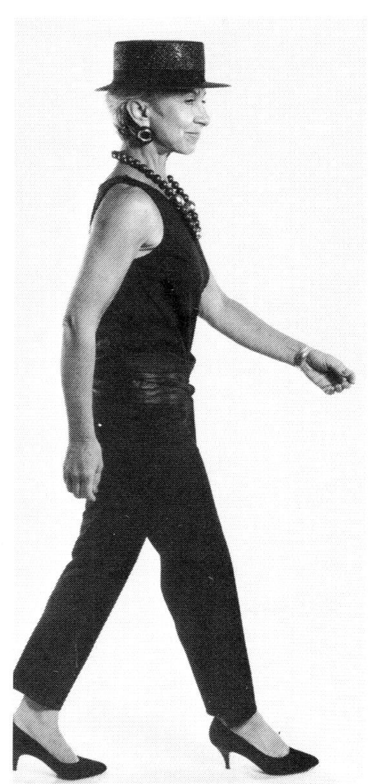
Right

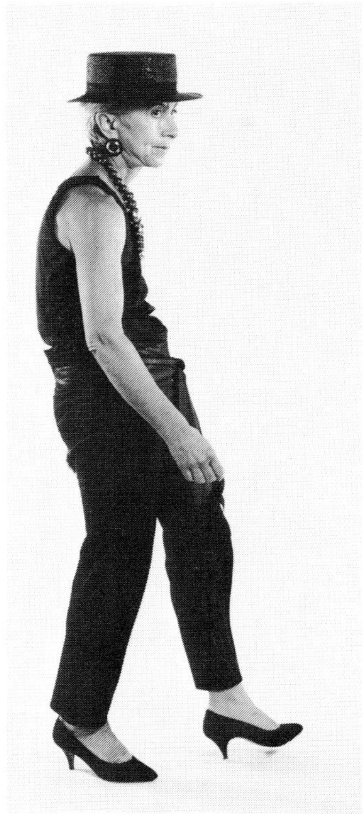
Wrong

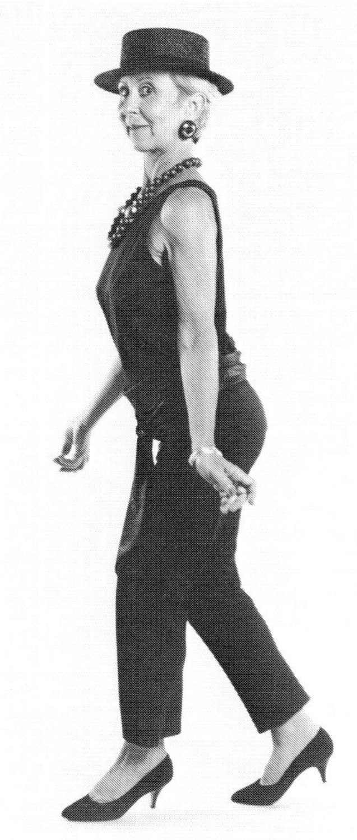
Wrong

STANDING IN HIGH HEELS

When you are standing in high heels, in either full or mini-alignment, the above instructions apply. Very high heels in either case, standing or walking, require you to accentuate the positive aspects of the Alignment even more, and do make sure, always, that you do not push your weight on to the joints of the big toes.

CARRYING SHOPPING BAGS

I have already mentioned dividing the load to be carried between two bags and how to carry them evenly along the sides of the torso. Remember that the shoulder rotation, up, back and down, should place the shoulder joints so that the shoulders are not rounded forward at all, otherwise they will be held in the out-of-line position by the weight of the bags.

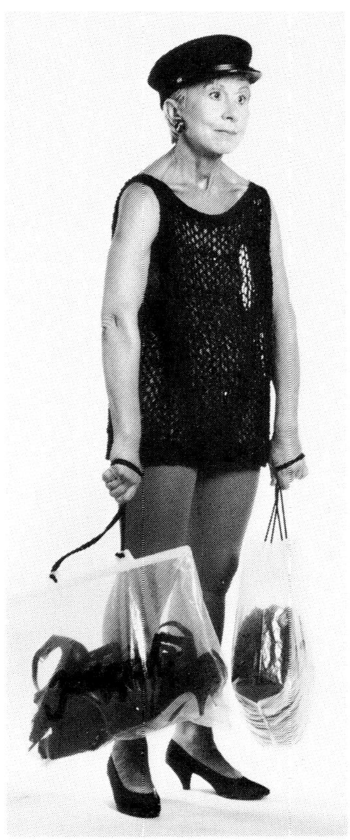

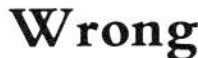

Wrong

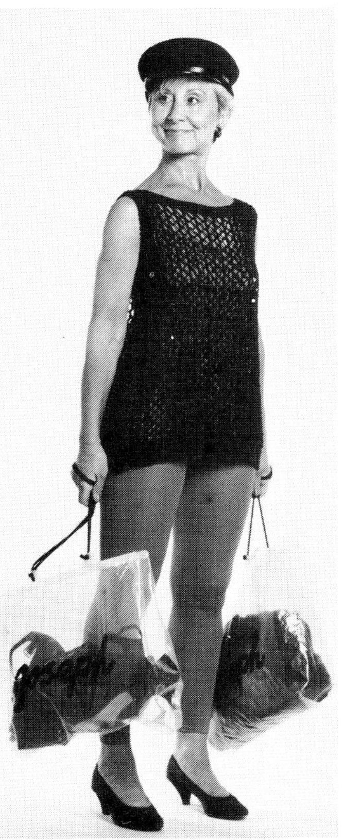

Right

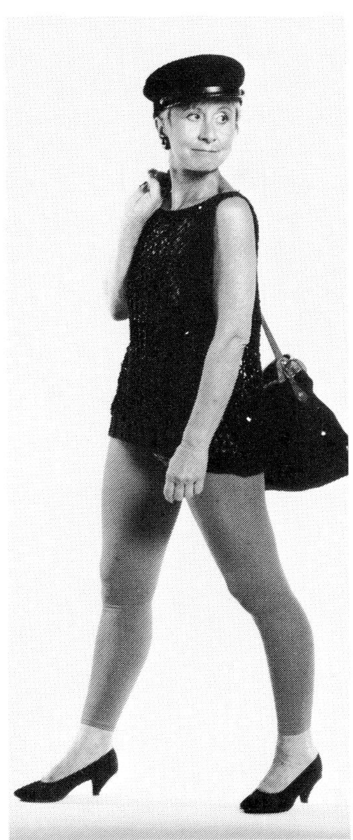

Right

Unfortunately, this is the manner – you can take a look at me doing it incorrectly – in which most people carry them. You can see how much it not only misaligns the shoulders but how the evidence of strain on the muscles of the neck and face cannot be avoided.

One bag can be slung over one shoulder and the handle held in your hand. Keeping the elbow down on that side ensures that you can even out the lateral line of the shoulders.

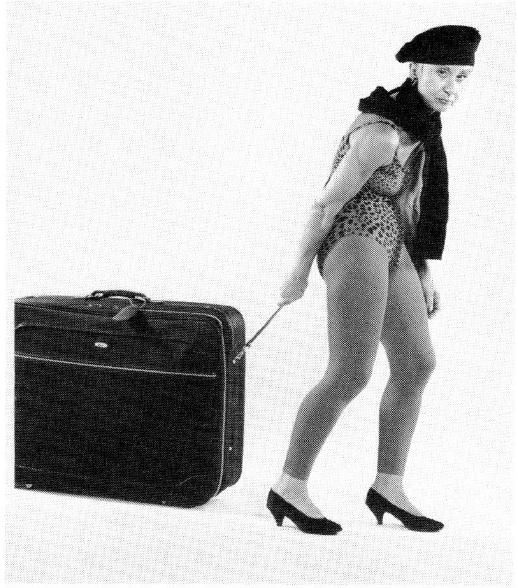

Wrong

PULLING SUITCASES – OR ANYTHING ELSE

Let your pulling arm extend back from the shoulder with the elbow straight. Try not to pull with the arm twisted, as this can put a strain on the hand-elbow-shoulder mechanism. Again, do not let the shoulder curve into a forward position, but keep it rotated down.

PUSHING

In the pictures of me in my role of homemaker/housekeeper I am doing the everyday task of carpet sweeping. This can be a push-and-pull motion. Keep your alignment going by doing a Knee Flex on the push, and when you pull back straighten or return into a straight-leg position. When you look at the floor, try not to extend your head forward but keep it back in line and drop the chin just enough so that the eyes can see down.

If you are pushing a lawn mower, or a pram, or a shopping cart, keep your body in a position so that the torso angles forward in the push from the hips. Do not curve your body over the handles, but maintain sufficient distance from the handles with your elbows flexed to stay aligned while you are pushing.

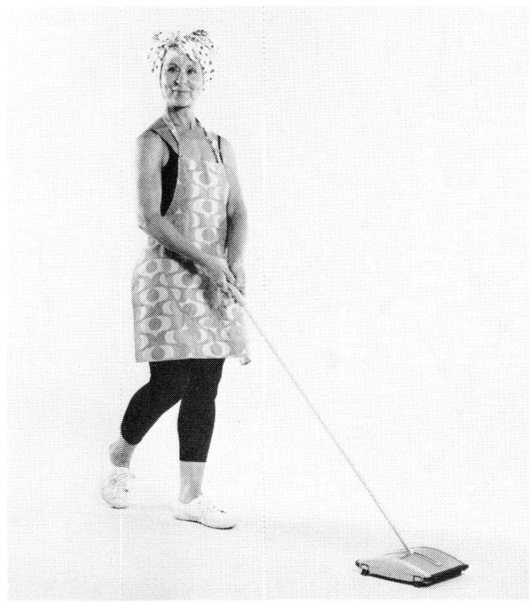

Right

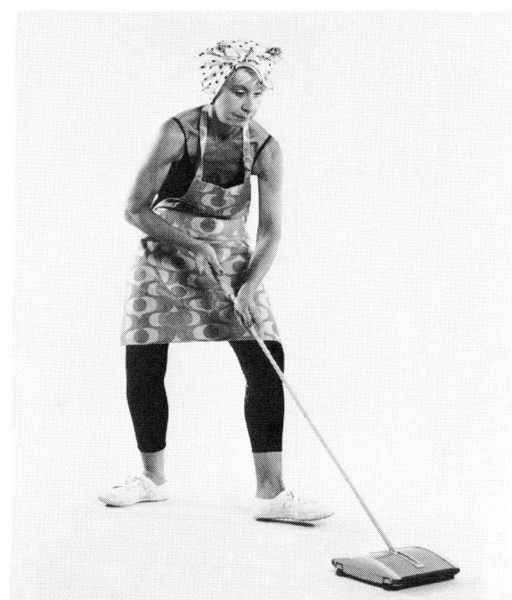

Wrong

RAISING YOUR ARMS

The number of times in a day we raise our arms, either from the elbow or from the shoulder, is uncountable. The joints and muscles involved in these movements are so complex and sophisticated we would probably remain immobilized were we aware what we were actually demanding of ourselves. Here are general rules for preserving the alignment benefits while using these complex procedures.

1. Keep your shoulders down and learn to use this ball-in-its-socket position as much as possible for movements that require the arm (whole or part) to be raised or rotated for reaching or holding.
2. Your elbows should be kept in line with your shoulders either alongside the torso when talking on the phone – see my picture – or when reaching upwards. The more

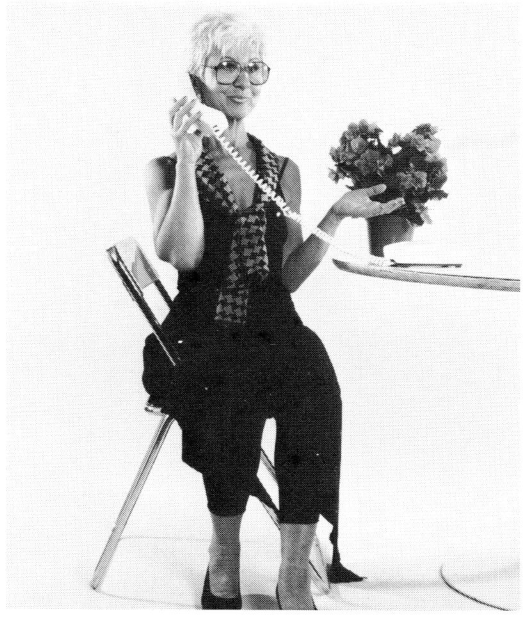

Right

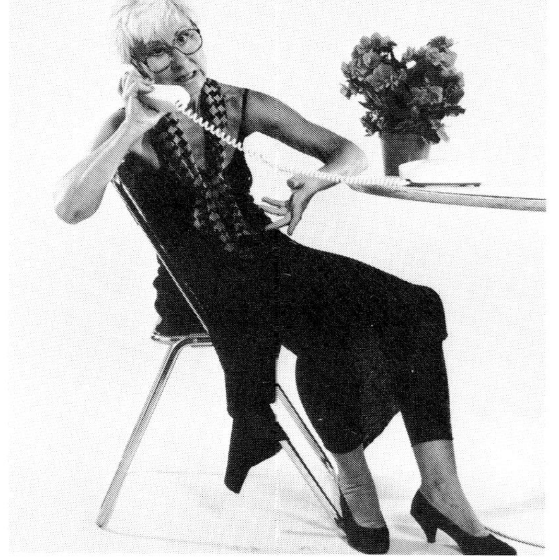

Wrong

you lift your arms by lifting your shoulder joints rather than keeping them down, the more you distort the alignment (especially the muscles in the neck) and daily acts become debilitating rather than remedial movements.

I have included my friend Andy doing his juggling act – something that is very difficult in a misaligned position. You may not have inclinations towards this particular profession, but it certainly proves the point about maximum manoeuvrability.

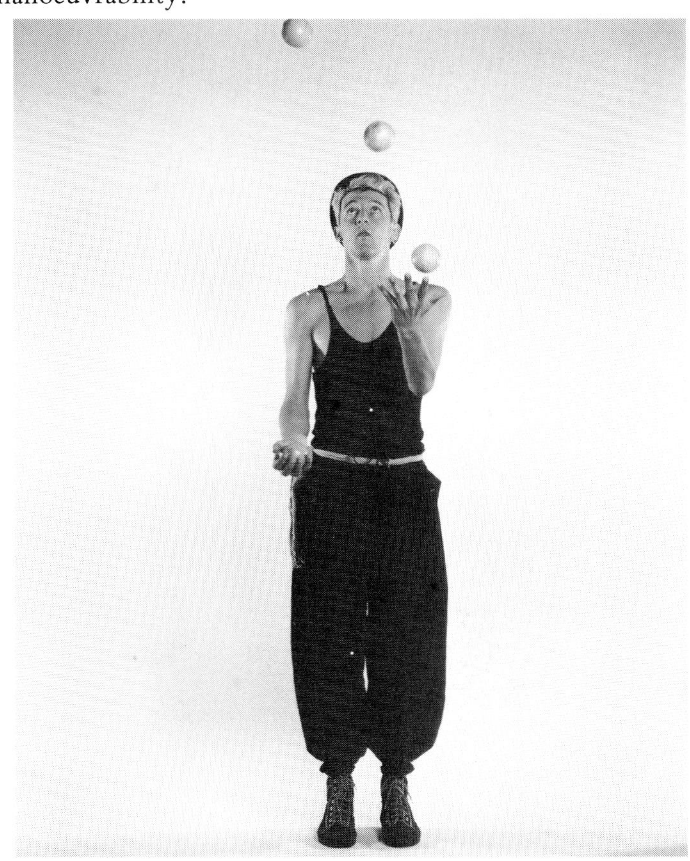

Right

There am I hailing a taxi – with genteel, cool, collected aligned demeanour – and there is the frightening apparition of me doing the same thing misaligned. The former obviously puts you in a more desirable position for overall body improvement, but I must admit that the latter, with its implication of demand and panic, may actually get the cab faster!

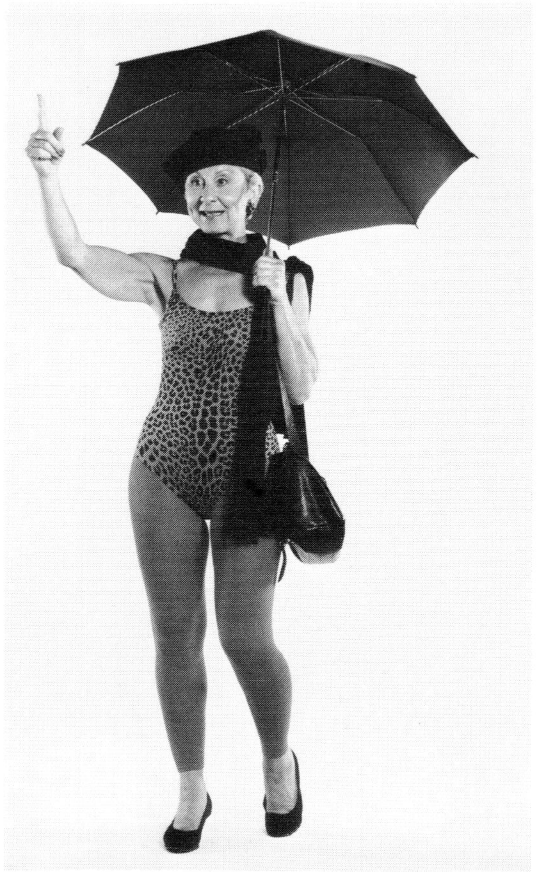

Right

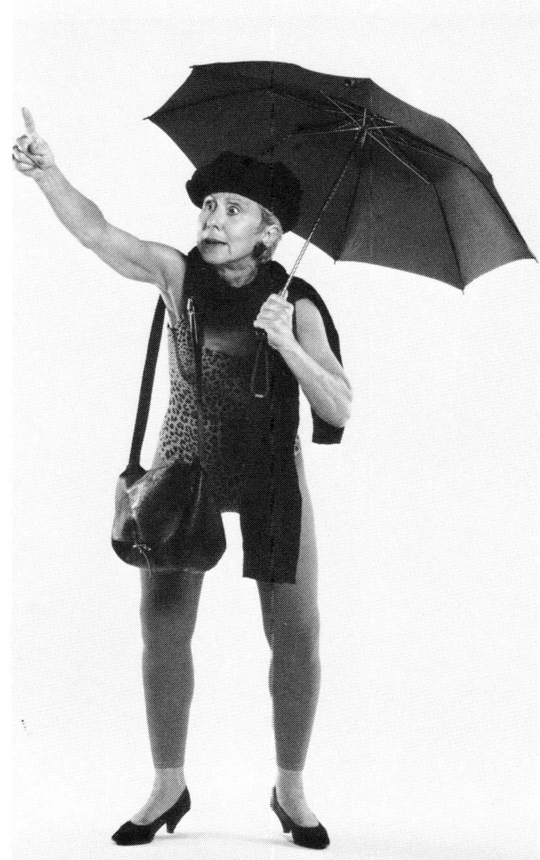

Wrong

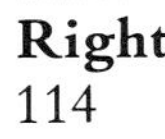

GOING UP AND DOWN STAIRS

Our acquaintance with Knee Flexes goes back to the instruction on how they are done in Section I. They are used in many movements in daily life and it is usually assumed that we can depend on our knees for the rest of our lives. If the knee joint is not exercised correctly, however, it is very likely to go wrong through injury and almost certainly to diminish in efficiency at a remarkably early stage. For evidence of this listen to people groan when they try to flex or bend their knees getting into chairs, and observe their need to 'pull' themselves upstairs. We use our elbows frequently in automatic flexing motions of opening and closing, but the knee joint is one we tend to keep fixed in either straight or flexed positions.

It should be exercised as a joint, and going up stairs, where it helps to lift the body weight, is an excellent time to use it. You can observe me in the 'right' pictures actually raising my body upwards in a vertical line by straightening my knee on each step *before* I place my other foot on the next step. The body aligned does not 'sit' heavily on the feet; it moves

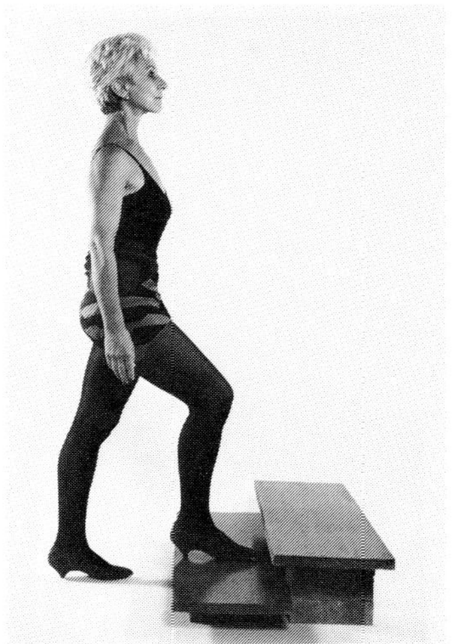

Right

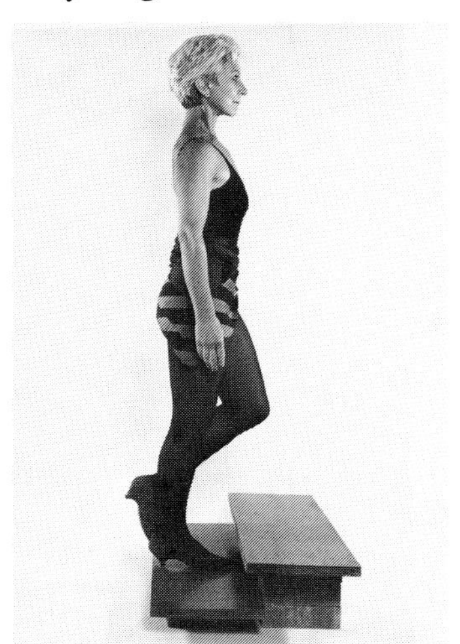

Right

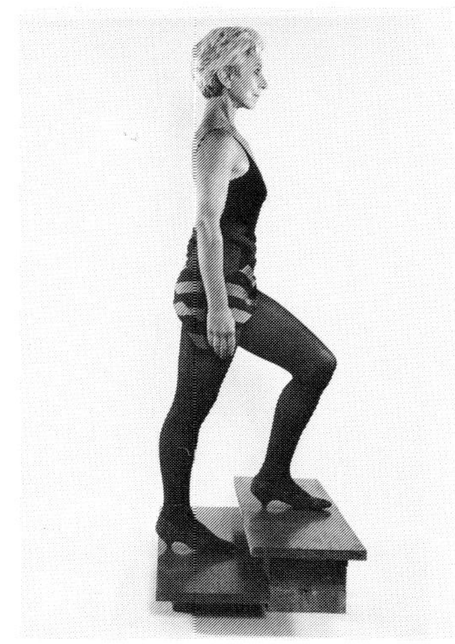

Right

straight up vertically and in this manner the knee joint is exercised without strain.

In the 'wrong' pictures you are able to see how not aligning, and not straightening the knee, creates an altogether lumbering and debilitating movement. If you hold on to a banister (and why not for balance?), see that you try not to use your hand in a pulling position in front of you, but as a balance only, at your side. With practice you'll be able to keep the body balanced with only a touch of the fingers. For those of you who have trouble with stairs because of arthritic or rheumatic conditions, take it easily, but try to do it, if only for a few steps and then a rest.

I must immodestly tell you that I can straighten my knees between each rise while I am running upstairs – but, then, I've been practising for thirty years!

When you descend, don't lean back but keep the body vertical and straighten your knee before you place your foot down on the next step. This can, when exaggerated, create that 'goose-step' look that you may wish to avoid, but done slowly and deliberately it can create an impression of cool self-possession and be most useful for those special occasions.

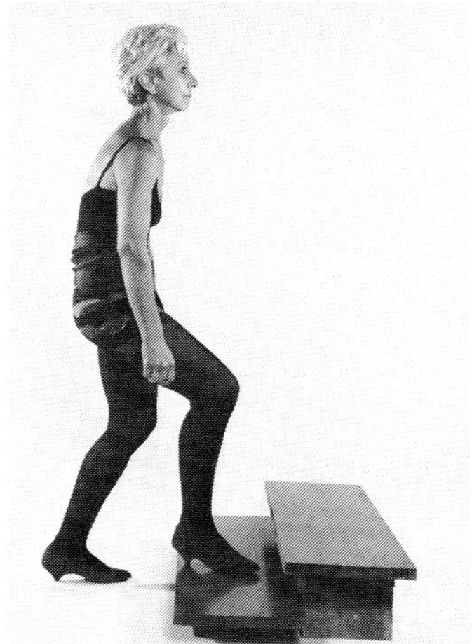

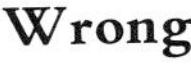

Wrong

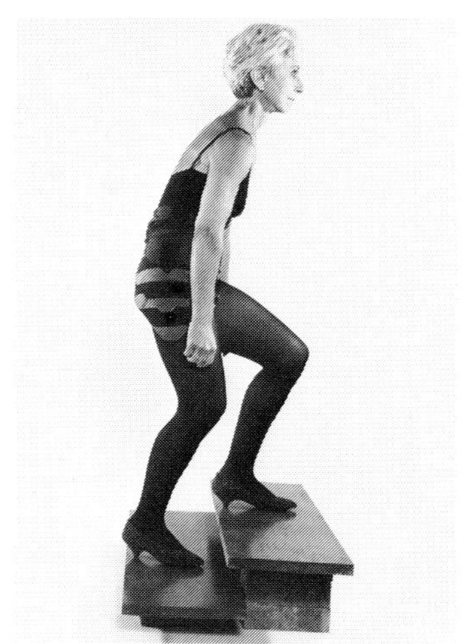

Wrong

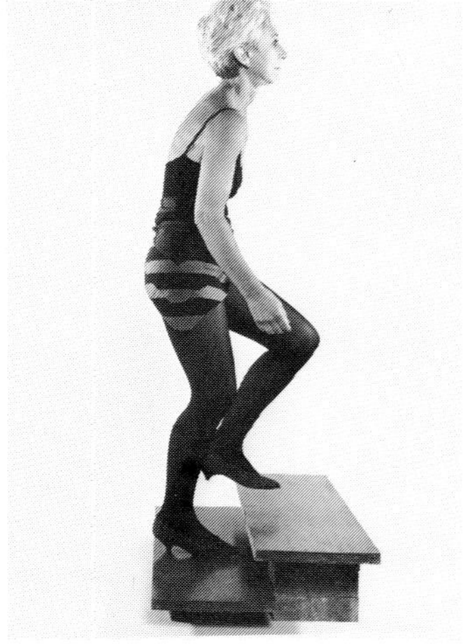

Wrong

THE HEEL RAISES

These help both in raising and lowering the body and can be used as beneficial movement if you keep your body aligned *as* you raise your heels. When you do raise them, try to keep in mind the triangles of the feet and the exact lines of balance over the insteps. Just as in walking in heels, the coccyx should be kept very well down with a good tightening into the front of the pelvis. Do not clench the cheeks of the buttocks but use the hip rotation to achieve this tightening.

Heel raises done on their own, for no other reasons except as an excellent means of developing balance, are invaluable. Get your body aligned and do a number in succession (raise your heels a quarter inch only). Don't pitch forward but use the same vertical line for movement up and down as described in the bounces.

BENDING AND LIFTING

For picking up heavy objects, first position your body so that your torso is aligned. Then do a Knee Flex, and raise your heels as you go down to take the strain off the leg muscles. Position yourself with your hands under the object and your elbows at your sides. As you lift, lower your heels, straighten your knees and keep your torso aligned as you come up. Andy can be seen doing it correctly in the picture sequence; we have no pictures of him doing it incorrectly, except in the preliminary stage, as our concern for his bodily welfare prevailed. You may notice that there are no pictures of me picking up heavy objects. It is something I avoid as often as possible. I would suggest you do the same, unless your work as a furniture dealer or a parent makes it unavoidable.

There is another way of lowering the body towards the ground and this is commonly called 'bending over'. Bending

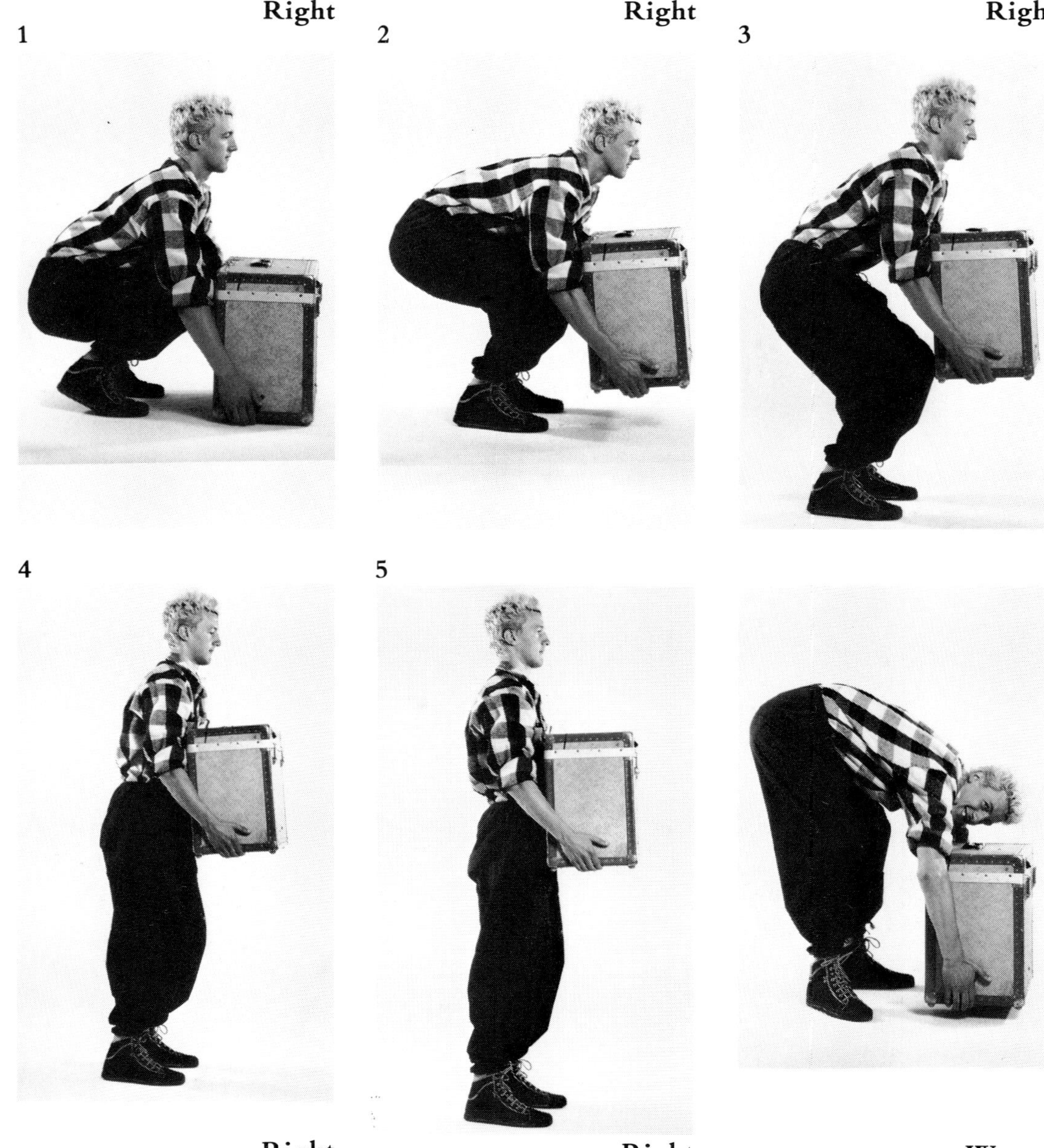
Right
1
Right
2
Right
3
4
5
Right
Right
Wrong

is difficult for the lower back if you go down by curving the spine, and even more troublesome and more likely to cause injury if you come up in this manner. Here is a stretch-without-strain way.

First align your body with your feet a bit wider apart than usual and make sure your hips are rotated into their abdominal tightening position. From the hips extend the entire torso, neck and head back in line straight towards the ground as you rotate your hips even more inwards. Do this slowly at first, extending your breastbone upwards, otherwise you will probably start caving in in the middle, which will mean a curving of the back. What you want to achieve is a long straight back stretch with the hip joints acting as the lowering and raising agents, not the lower back.

You can, if you are sufficiently flexible, use this movement to get your torso far enough down towards the ground to pick up something light, or, if your hamstrings are too tight for this (as is the case with about 90% of the population), do a

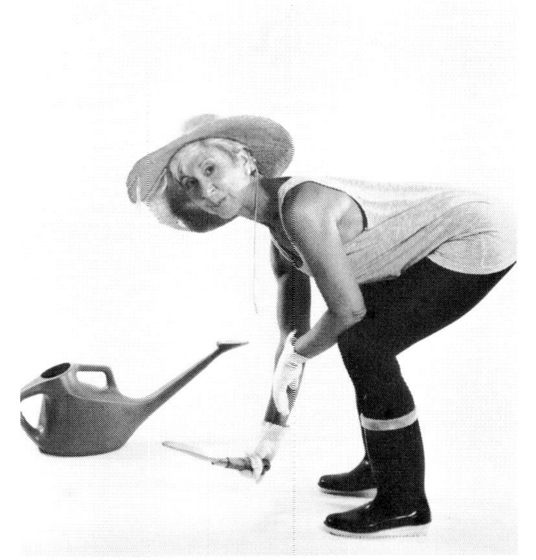

Right

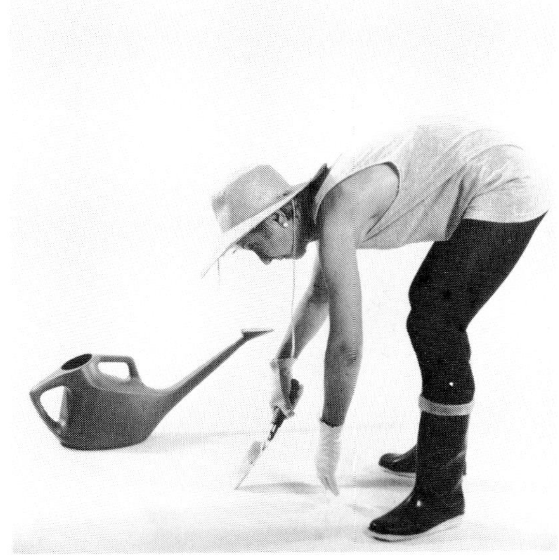

Wrong

Knee Flex as soon as you feel them pull, and support your back by placing your elbows on the tops of your knee-caps with your hands hanging between. You are then in an aligned, supported position, and with one hand you can pick things up, weed the garden, or whatever. No strain – even in the face! You can see me doing this in the garden, or *almost* in the garden, pictures.

When you come up, place your hands over the tops of your knee-caps, elbows in at the sides of your torso, then straighten your knees first. After this, move your torso up to a vertical position from your hips keeping the crown-of-head-to-coccyx line absolutely straight – just like a see-saw. As the head comes up the coccyx moves into its 'down position'.

If you have lowered your torso without the Knee Flex, come up in exactly this same balanced way.

If you are making a bed, or talking to a child or looking for a four-leaf clover, you can use either one or a combination of all these for getting down to it.

SITTING

Sitting may rest your legs, but done incorrectly and over a sustained period of time it can be extremely hard on the back, and getting in and out of chairs is in fact a gymnastic accomplishment in itself.

The reason sitting is a difficult position to maintain satisfactorily is quite straightforward. Your spine, flexible by design, must be strong enough to hold up vertically without the additional support of your legs. So chairs were created to make it easier, and a lot of help they have been for the most part! Recently some thoughtful people have started designing chairs that have putative therapeutic value. They are intended to position the body in ways that help to relieve the strains other chairs create. However, my thinking, consistent and predictable, is that your own body, positioned correctly by you, is the only overall solution to remedying the problem. In the first place, it is difficult to carry the right chair around with you all the time.

To my way of thinking (I'm five foot three), no one has ever made a 'comfortable chair' comfortable. For me, basic straight-backed chairs are far better.

WATCHING TV

Posing for these photographs, Andy and I were truly an odd couple. I was the one who decided that in the pictures I would be right and he would be wrong. After all, I am thirty-seven years older than he, and equal rights can be taken just so far! As you can see, youth and age can be juxtaposed in many ways if the self-image is secure enough!

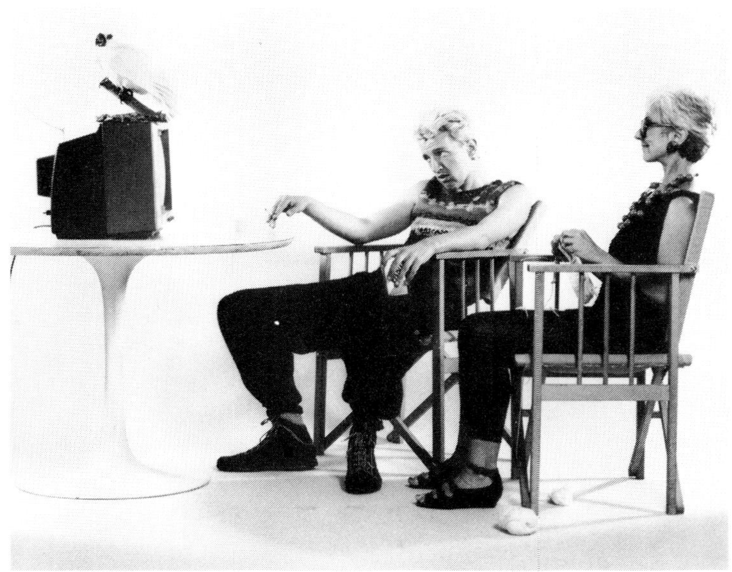

IN THE EXECUTIVE CHAIR

In these pictures, you can see very clearly how a curved back indicates strain, stress and age, and a straightened back gives an image of ease, control and agelessness. Most training courses and magazines have pushed the importance of body language in a business context, and most executives are aware of it. You should be able to indicate, for example, interest and involvement by moving towards someone, or, conversely, a distancing from demands or discussion by moving the body away. Correct body alignment will let you use your body as you wish – or as indicated by a particular situation. It is pointless to speak of body behaviour if the body is not supple enough to do it.

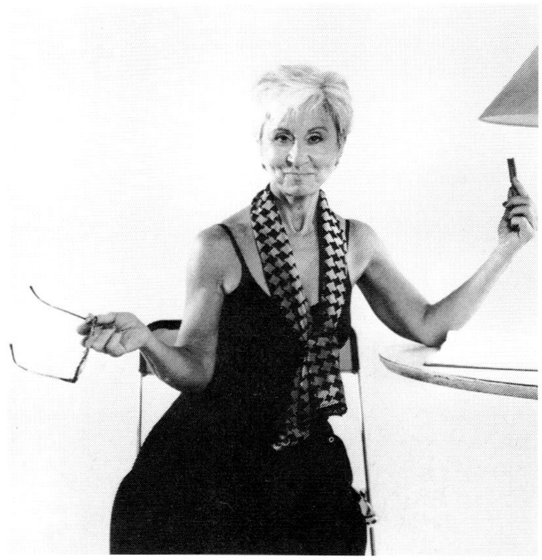

Right

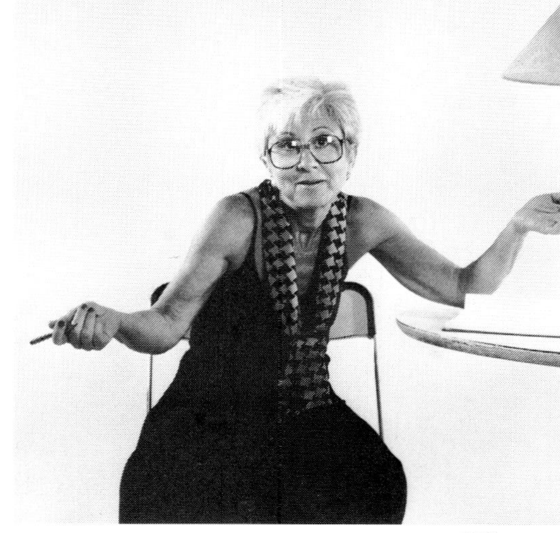

Wrong

MAKE-UP

Seeing those pictures was, even for me, a startling and revealing experience. The differences you can see are merely the differences between alignment and misalignment. The way I maintained the alignment was primarily by bringing the mirror towards me. We could learn to do this in many situations – reading, writing, shaving the face (get a mirror where you won't have to strain to look into it), eating, and so on. (While we are on the subject of eating, imagine – in fact, don't imagine, experiment right now – how much better for your jaws and facial muscles it is to chew with your head back in line rather than chewing with your chin jutting forwards.)

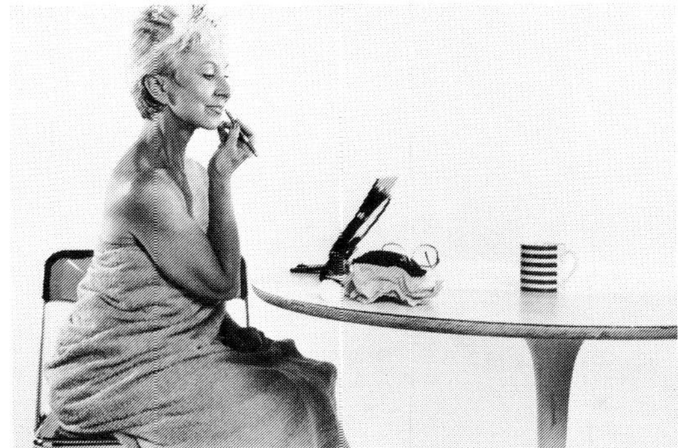

Right

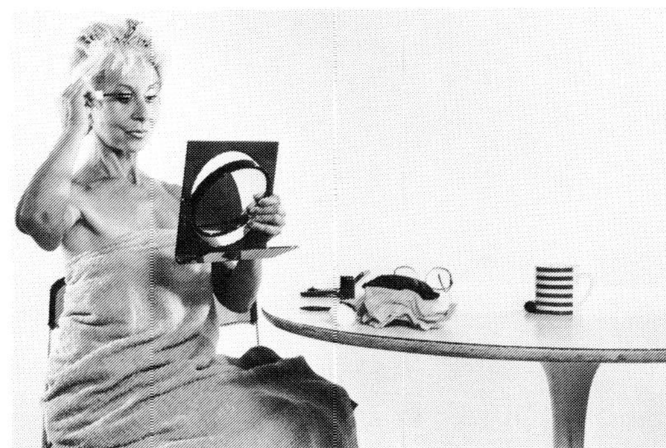

Right

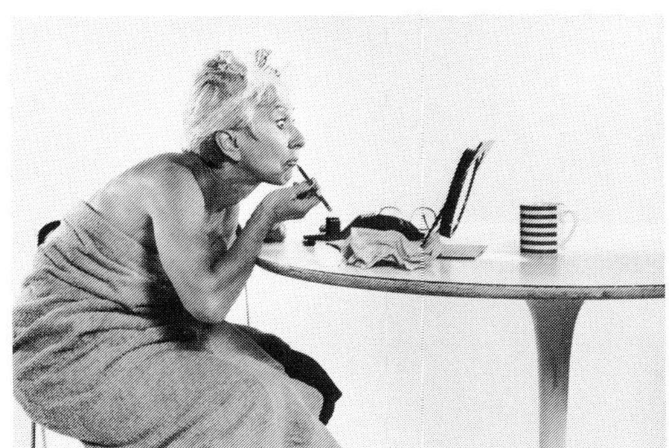

Wrong

TYING YOUR SHOE LACE

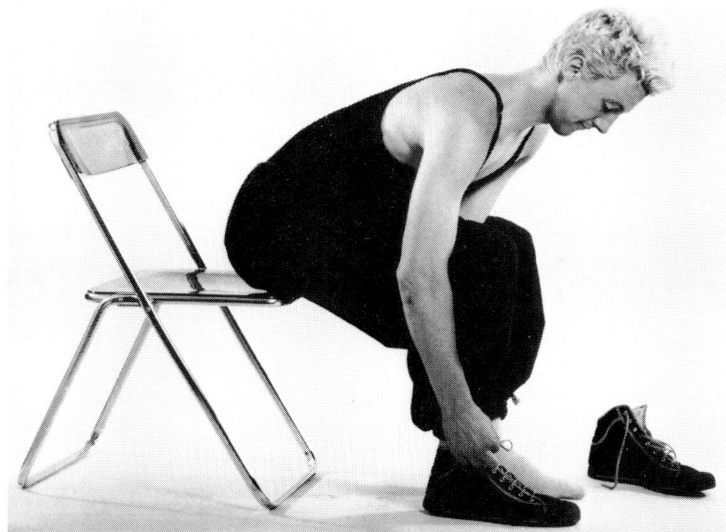

Right

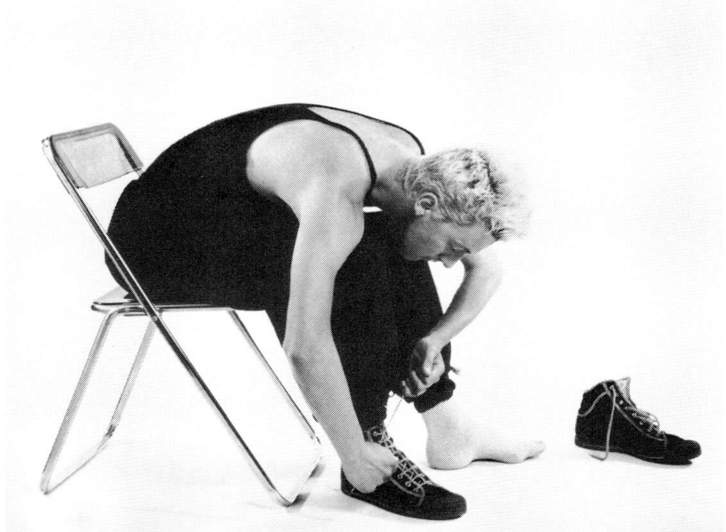

Wrong

Even if you are tall, like Andy, and feel you can reach over to tie your shoe, you will still be putting your body in a curved position. Instead, position yourself towards the edge of the chair and keep your foot in an aligned position under the knee. Extend your torso from the hip joints, so that your spine can stretch across your thighs, your shoulders remain down and your neck and head free. Remember, throughout everything, that lifted shoulders tighten and restrict neck muscles, and that is precisely what makes them painful. When you raise the torso up from this position, return as you went down with the spine straight from the hip joints. Of course, your coccyx remains down in line with the 'sitting bones', and you remember to keep tightening the lower abdomen.

TURNING YOUR HEAD

One of the observations often made by ageing motorists is of the increasing and apparent difficulty in being able to turn the head when reversing the car. Indeed, the contortionist positions often adopted to do the job defy description. I am going to give you some minor instructions with very positive results so that you can continue turning your head rather than tilting it from side to side.

First make sure you are fully aligned sitting in a chair.

Visualize your head as the world (we are thinking big!), and your neck as a vertical *axis*. Slowly rotate your head to the right keeping the crown of your head back in line with your neck. The left side of your chin will probably lift upwards as you turn – keep it very well down and do not let it jut forward. Keep your shoulders down. You should feel a slight pull in the right side of your neck down to the right shoulder. Stop when you cannot turn any more without tilting the left side of your chin upwards. Slowly turn your head back to the forward position. Re-align, and do the same rotation to the left, keeping the right side of your chin down.

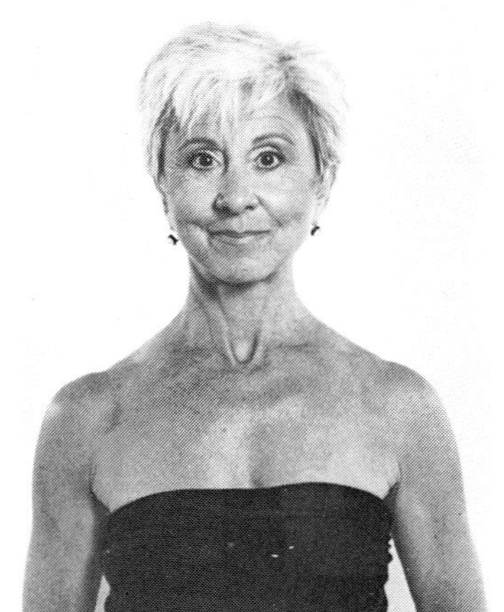

Right

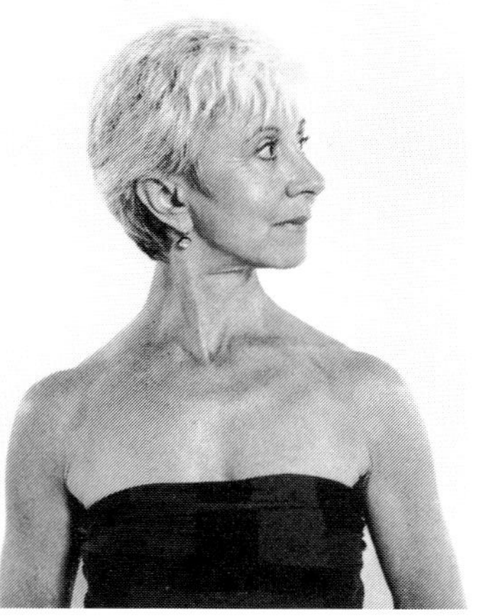

Right

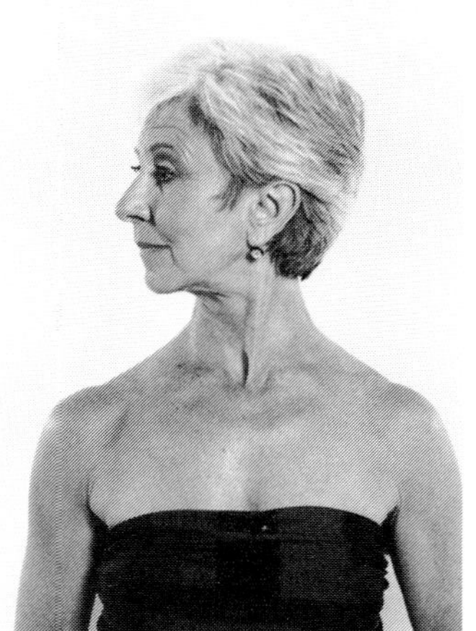

Right

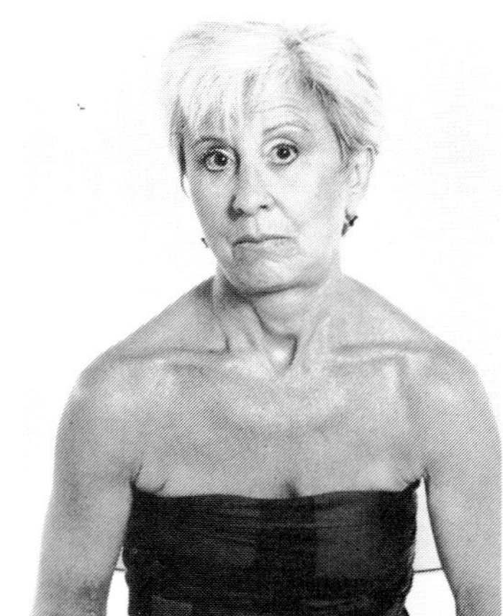

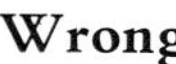

Wrong

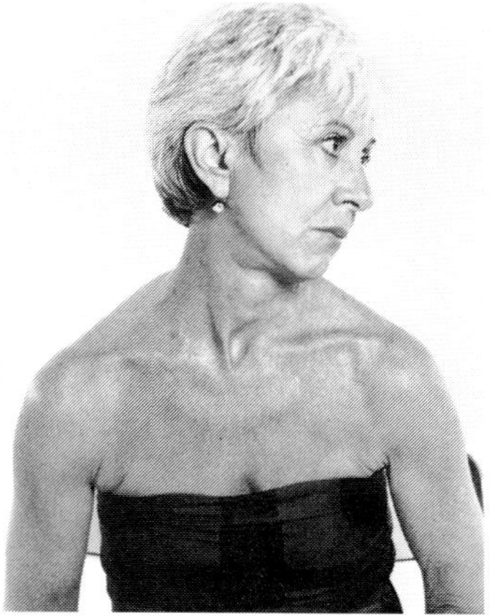

Wrong

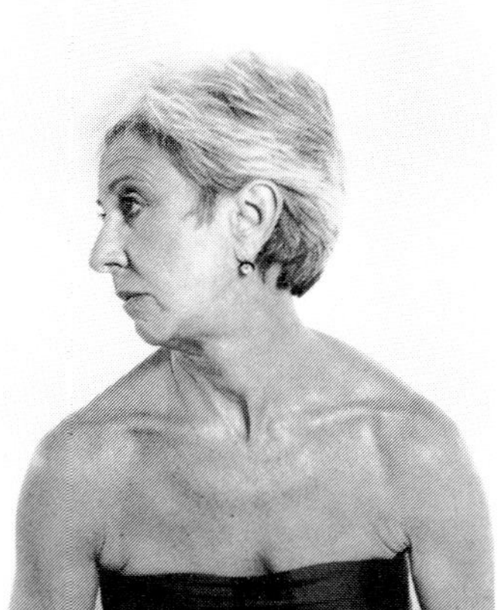

Wrong

It is the head-back-in-the-line-with-the-spine that permits this rotation and approximates the positions achieved through manipulation.

It is very common to have no real idea of how your body is positioned other than by observing it in a mirror. Generally we have no experience of feel-memory in ourselves and must continually refer to mirrors for affirmation of how our bodies look and are positioned. This often results in delusions about reality and these head turns are a case in point. When I teach them to people, they almost invariably tilt their heads to the side but are honestly convinced they are turning them. To remedy this and to achieve the desired results I suggest, as we did in the Triangles, use the mirror first and make adjustments to achieve the corrected position; then very consciously register the feel. This is an ideal time to use your Triangle shoulder-points as guides for direction.

To use the mirror in the head turns (think of them as rotations on a vertical axis), stand in profile to a mirror that reflects your head and shoulders. Slowly rotate your head towards the mirror until you feel a definite but tolerable pull along the sides of the neck. As you do this, and when you stop, your chin line should be parallel to the collar-bone line – exactly like the Triangle line-up. Look at your reflection in the mirror. Be sure your face is straight and not tilted or slanted to the side. Correct it if necessary, close your eyes and register the feel.

Face the other direction for the opposite turn. Here is an interesting experiment to validate the effectiveness of correct alignment. When you have rotated your head as far as it will go, feeling a tolerable pull, stop. Then do one more shoulder rotation very precisely – up, back and down. You will probably find that this will give you the additional stretch needed to rotate your head even more.

Use these head turns whenever your neck is feeling tight and strained – two or three rotations from side to side, done quite slowly, is about the right number. Finish up with a longer-than-usual Release, and a good explosive A-A-A-H-H-H-H-H-H-H-H Stretch.

The head turns can be practised when looking from side to side for oncoming traffic when driving, waiting to cross a street on foot, or getting the most from the finals at Wimbledon. Turning your head correctly will make all these movements more effective.

GETTING INTO A CHAIR

Since sitting in a chair also involves the procedures of getting into and out of it, here is my advice on the whole subject.

1. Make sure your Mini-Aligned body is positioned so that the backs of your heels are not too far away from the front legs of the chair.
2. Start your sitting movement with a Knee Flex, and, as you lower your body towards the seat of the chair, move your torso slightly forwards from the hips, keeping your back straight.
3. When your bottom reaches the edge of the seat, your torso should still be in its slightly diagonal straight line and your hands should be placed on the chair seat alongside your hips for balance and support.

You are now, once more, on the edge of your chair and it is not at all a bad place to be. Sitting back in a soft chair almost inevitably means having to fight a slump in the lower back, and sitting in an aligned and upright position on the edge of a chair can be surprisingly comfortable. Try it! However, if you want to move back into the chair, use your hands for support and lift your bottom slightly off the seat. Move the entire torso backwards, keeping your spine straight, until the 'sitting bones' are placed in the rear of the seat. Keep those abdominal muscles tight throughout and do not allow the lower back to curve.

Straighten your body from the hips into a vertical sitting position, mini-align again – and there you are!

Right

Right

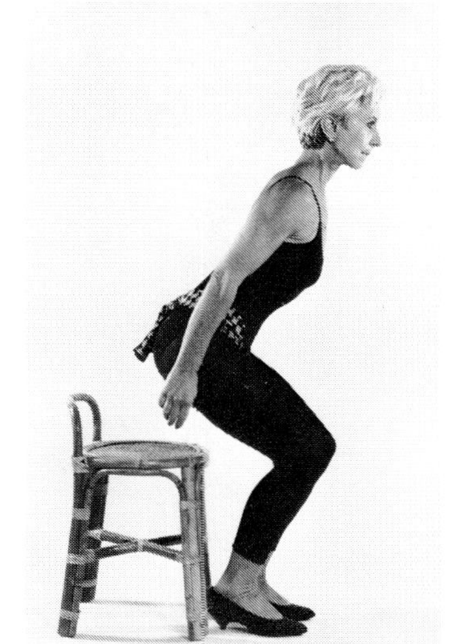

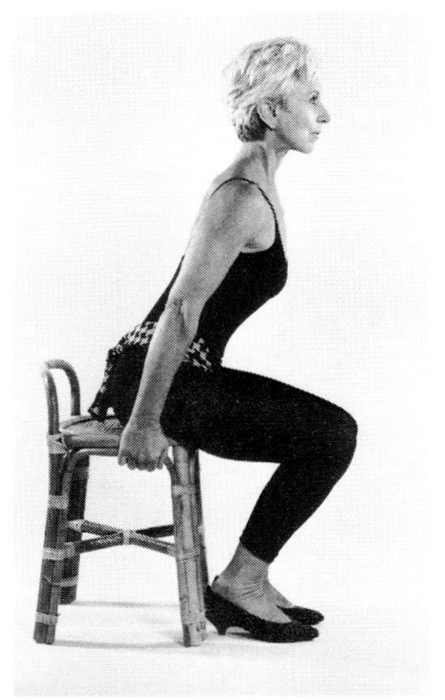

Right

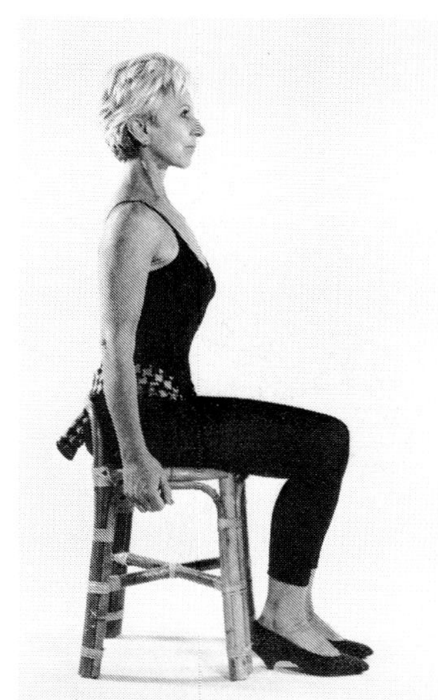

Right

Wrong

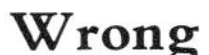

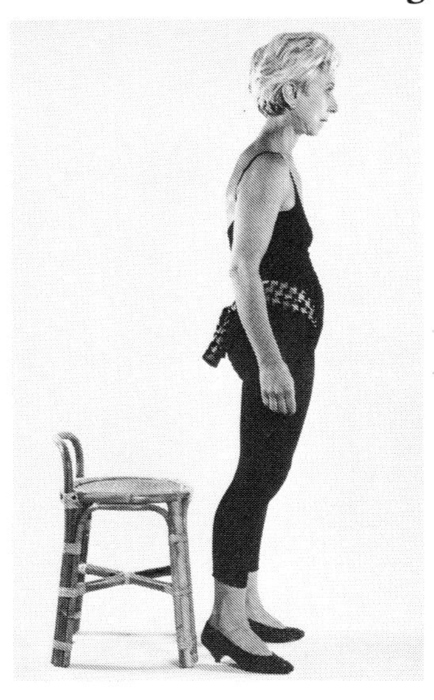

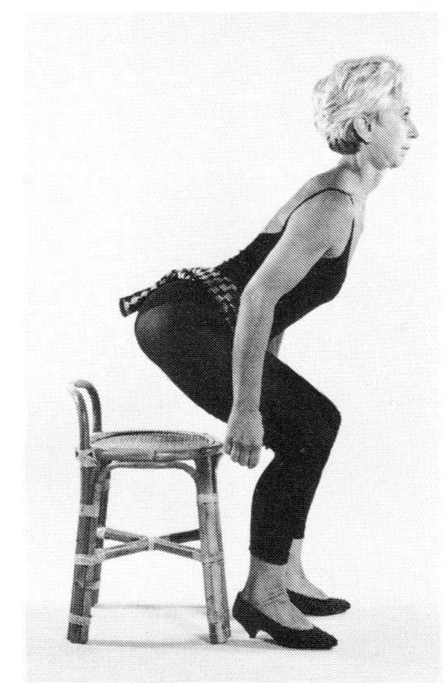

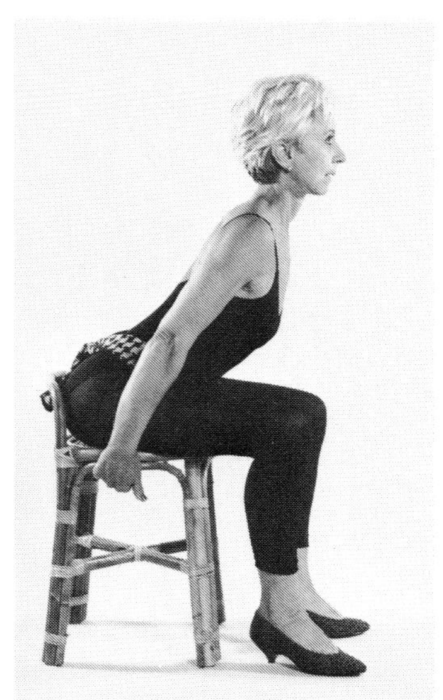

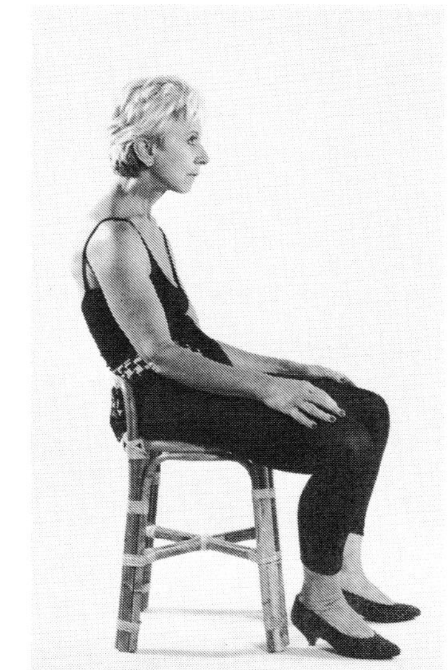

Wrong

Wrong

SOME ADVICE ON SITTING

1. Keep your feet directed forward (even if you cross them).
2. Make sure you keep those lower abdominal muscles really tight in order to support your lower back.
3. Keep your head back in its mini-aligned position.

These three points ensure that both ends are right and what comes in the middle is supported.

Try to avoid:

1. Backing into a chair – that means starting so far away you must sit down by arching your lower back and leading with your bottom.
2. Sitting down in one movement – this almost guarantees you will have to use your 'backing in' position throughout. You simply won't be able to manoeuvre it any other way, and it also means you are more apt to 'fall' into the chair.

If you do approach sitting down by 'backing in', you will probably 'slump' your body immediately into a curved-forward position to try to relieve the strain you have just put on your lower back by leading with your bottom. Incidentally, once you are seated, and aligned, using pillows or cushions for support when the chair isn't doing the job is a very good idea. They are not, when you are aligned, being used to prop you up – they are for support only.

GETTING OUT AND UP FROM A CHAIR

This is simply a reversal in movements of those describing how to get down and into a chair. (One might as well accept, however, that nothing will be simple about extricating oneself from a comfortable seductive sofa.) Remember to use your hands close to the sides of your hips to lift your torso up and forward to the edge of the chair and to help get you into a standing position. (The arms of the chair can help but try to position your hands so they are only a bit in front of the shoulder line.) All movements should be made with your spine as straight as possible and a good strong tightening of the muscles into the front of the abdomen.

Of course there are exceptions to all rules. For instance, a mad dash from your seat to make it through an automatic door, or a quick goodbye from a back-seat pass, may mean you will have to sacrifice positioning for effective exiting. But just remember that fast, uncalculated movements can create fast, uncalculated injuries.

SPORTS

Let me explain straight away that a lot of my sporting life these days is restricted to rolling the ball at the end of my knitting yarn – or, better still, watching the cat do it! However, at one point I did play tennis and was passably good, I did ski and was very good, and I even went so far in golf as to marry a scratch player.

So when you look at these sports pictures of me you can be assured that 'right' and 'wrong' are to do with body alignment and certainly not to do with any developed expertise. I am demonstrating how by misalignment you can put your body into some really unattractive and potentially damaging positions, and then, by using the same situations – and the same body – with alignment, turn wrong into right and negative into positive.

The aligned body position quite evidently improves the quality of sports activity whether the participants are amateurs or professionals. First and foremost is improvement in perfor-

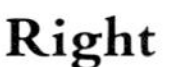

Right

Wrong

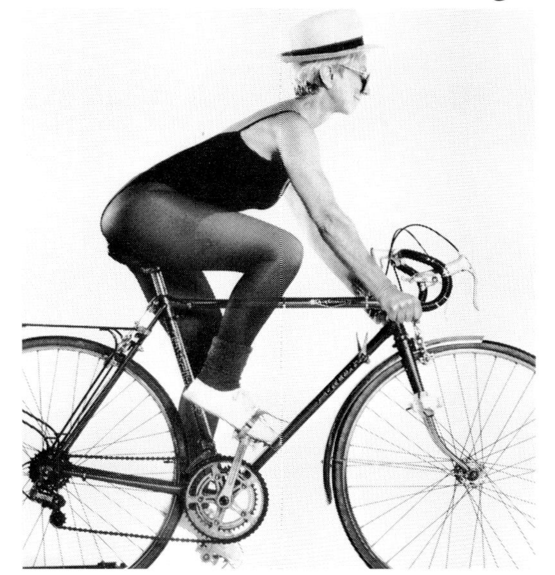

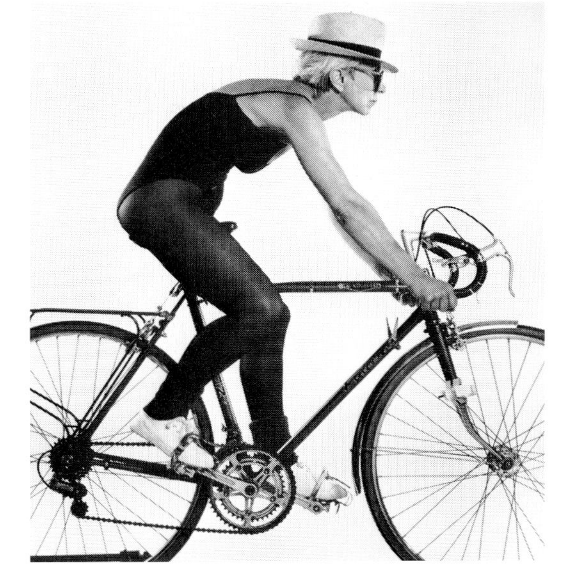

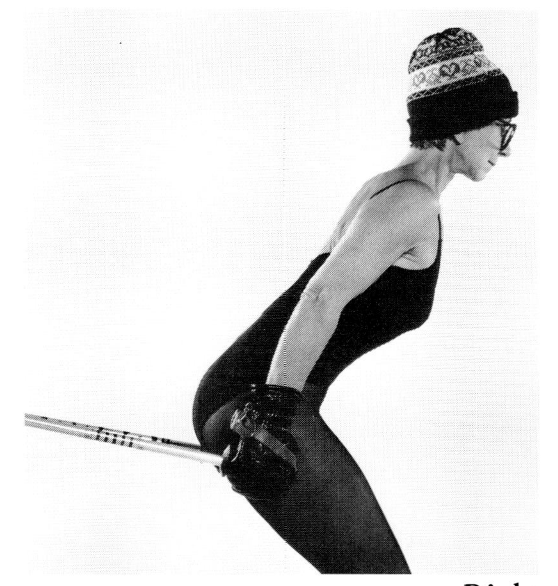

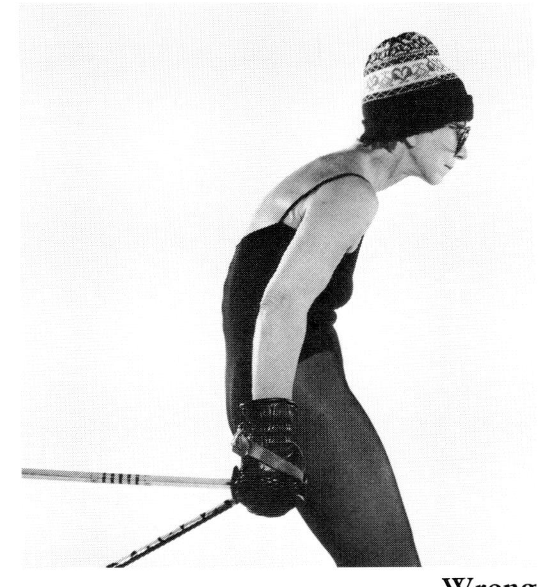

Right

Wrong

Right

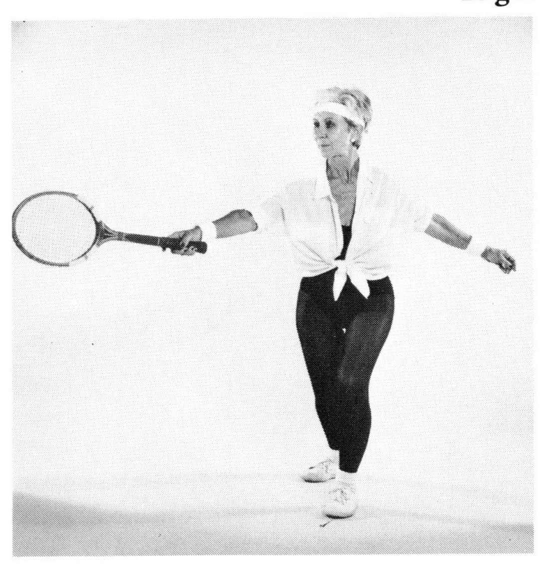

Wrong

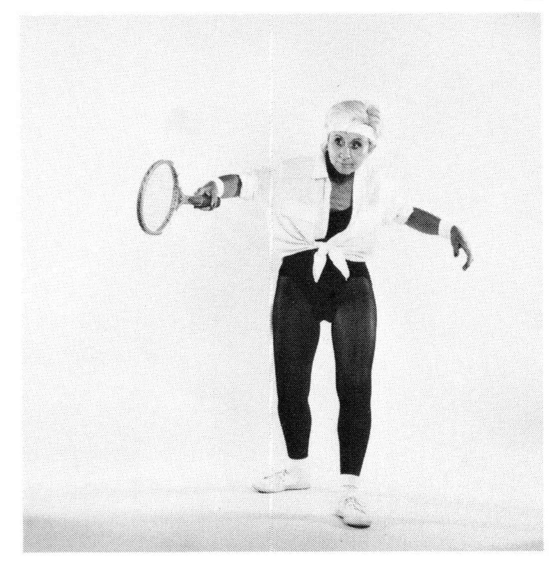

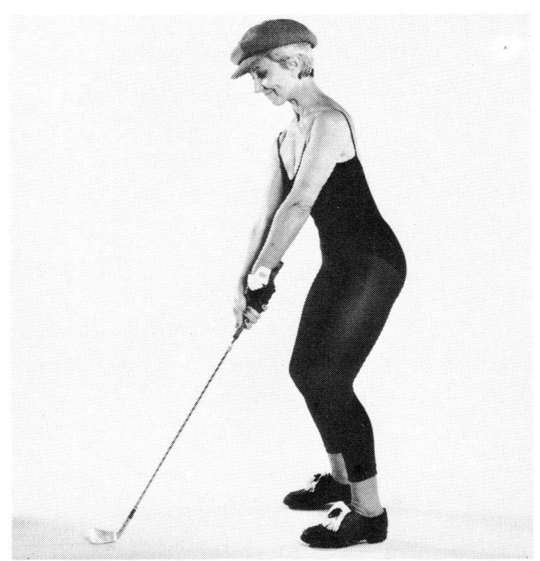

Right

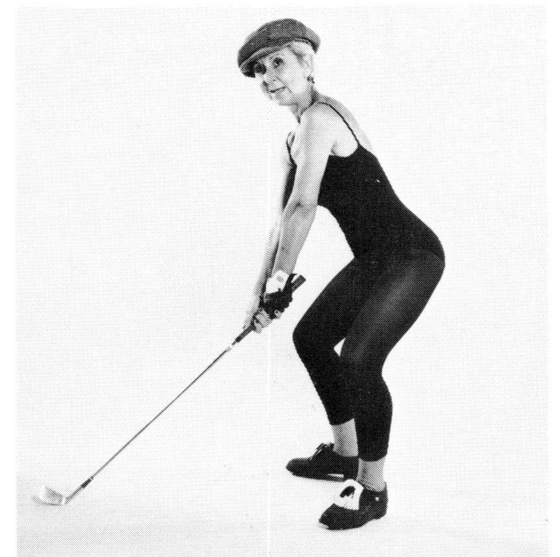

Wrong

mance. Correct alignment affords you much greater flexibility and all movements become more efficient and easier – the prerequisites of successful sports participation. The marvellous part is that positive effects take place as you are enjoying the sport, and improvements become apparent without your even being aware that they are taking place.

I had a pupil in California who, among other impressive achievements, was a cracking good amateur tennis player. She had a background of the very best instruction and exposure to the game, as she was the daughter of probably the most highly respected tennis journalist of that time (or perhaps of all time). One night after dinner at her home (she had been using the alignment for about a year) I asked her how her game was. She replied, 'My God, I'm glad you brought that up, I've been meaning to ring you to tell you something! You know I was really pleased when the stiffness in my finger joints got better [she was a concert pianist and had primarily been interested in the Alignment to help with that] but what I hadn't anticipated was the incredible change it has made in my tennis!' She went on to say that her service had never been really strong enough, but that the shoulder rotations the Alignment requires had obviously loosened those joints and positioned them so that the muscles' stretch and strength were able to work to much greater advantage. Her service had become so strong and reliable that, she went on to say, 'had this happened earlier I probably would have made it to Forest Hills'.

As efficiency increases through use of the Alignment, the aches and pains concomitant with the body-machine working out of line decrease. The muscle-build becomes an insurance policy in itself. One of my pupils came to me because of a lower-back problem – an avid golfer with a neurotic drive (both ways!). He found that by learning how to use his feet correctly and relating this to the positioning of his hip joints and pelvis he not only got rid of his back-ache but put fifty more yards on his drive.

Another pupil, a lady who swam every day, used only the

back-stroke and complained of continual neck pains. I suggested she concentrate on the part of the Alignment that raises the breastbone while she was back-stroking. In doing this her neck was freed of tension and pain and she became the outstanding style-setter on Ladies' Day at the swimming club!

Don't go away to try it all out yet – this last example is of an amateur rugby player who attributed new understanding and super-improvement in execution to having learned the power-principle of the Alignment and using it in kicking the ball (from the hips, not the lower back). I congratulated him on his success and asked him, 'Where to from here?' He looked dreamy and said, 'Who knows, perhaps I'll. . . .' I've never found out if he left his bank job or not – but open options are certainly wonderful to contemplate.

For those people who do not really want to be sports players, but who want to look good and play around the edges of sports, the Alignment is a must. The body will be well balanced, will look well shaped – taut and fit – and, because you will have learned and decided to use your body in a way that is best for you, self-confidence will be so apparent that you should be able to knock 'em over without even having to move out of the shade!

There is undoubtedly some value to a kind of exercise that is currently known as 'aerobic'. The word, however, has been thrown around and bent out of shape (as have many of the people who have worked in it) to the extent that its definition has become in many cases both ridiculous and dangerous.

The principal definition for the word 'aerobic' in *Collins English Dictionary* is 'depending on free oxygen or air'. The secondary definition is 'of, or relating to aerobes'. So let us look at 'aerobes'.

Definition: 'an organism that requires free oxygen or air'.

In other words, *me* and *thee*, and the entire human race. Every movement we make *is aerobic*.

Energetic movement, it has been fairly well established, is desirable in order to exercise the heart. It aids in helping it to function better and, hopefully, longer. However, if this kind of movement (fast and continuous) is not developed in a gradual way, and is over-done, there is powerful evidence that a great deal of harm can result – not just to the heart but to all the organs.

Right

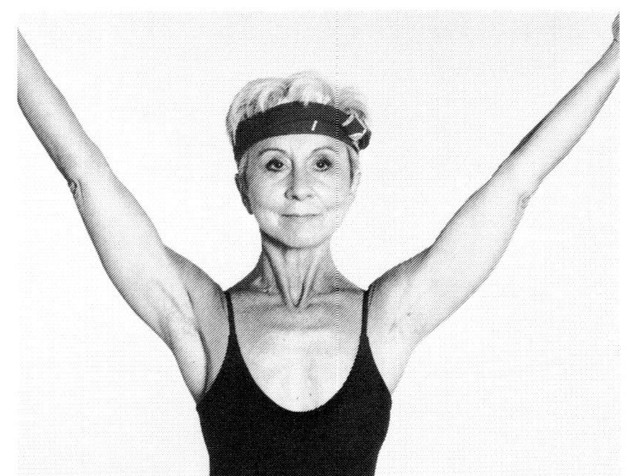

Wrong

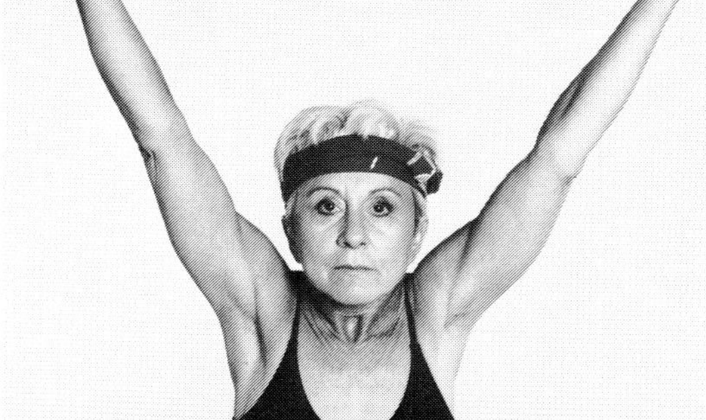

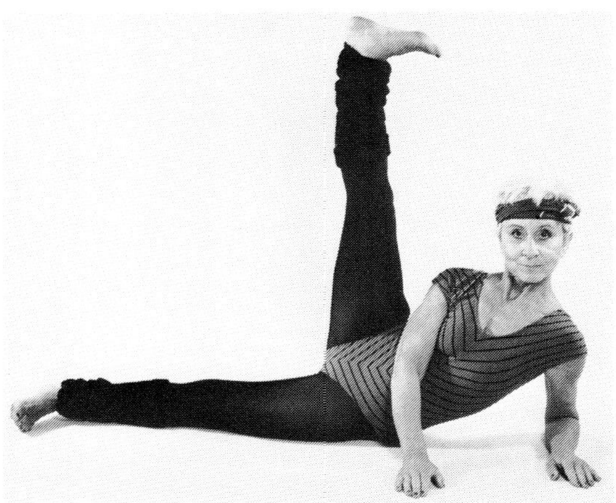

Right

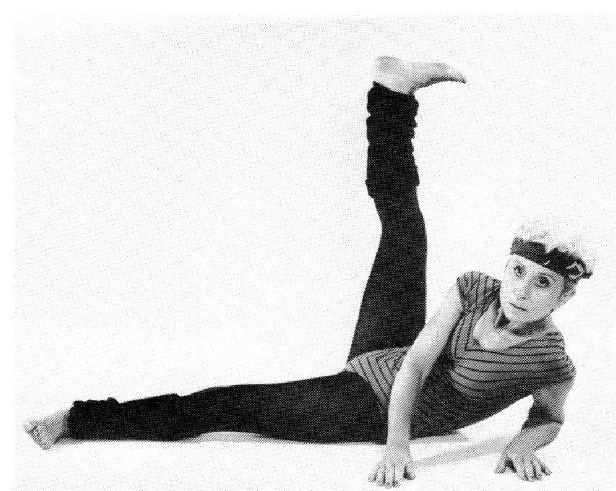

Wrong

ment assists in the effectiveness of almost all exercise, individual self-assessment is the important guide.

Do not be persuaded into programmes of any kind because of images other people have created for themselves. Those designed for top athletes, dancers and exercise fanatics – professional and amateur – may not be for you. Look at your personal needs. Assess yourself as honestly as possible, and ask questions. Look at and listen to the people who are giving you the answers. Think. Use your common sense. Chronological age is not the determinant but your individual condition, physically and emotionally.

A PREGNANT THOUGHT

Very little consideration is given to teaching women how to carry their infants before they are born. Some very thoughtful and intelligent people have made wonderful contributions on the subject of how to achieve healthy and happy pregnancies. Relaxation techniques, exercise manuals, advice of almost every kind proliferates and there have been some enlightened breakthroughs in many areas. However, I have yet to see anything that actually shows a pregnant woman how to position her feet so that she is 'carrying' rather than 'dropping' in her pregnancy, and how that relates to the inevitable backache.

Let us simplify this.

Right now, you are not pregnant. We shall assume you have stood, sat, walked and so on all your life with your feet in a slanted-out, ankles-pushed-in, incorrect position. This position has opened your pelvis outwards so that your lower abdominal muscles are out and down, rather than up and in. In turn, because what happens in the front affects what happens in the back, and vice versa, this has put a curve in your lower back. You are (and have been) classically misaligned.

You now become pregnant. What happens? You put the extra weight and strain of the baby into the area that is already out and down – and this weight and strain increases, for nine months. As the front goes out and down, the back curves in more and more – and you think you can escape a backache? All of this puts pressure down on to those poor flattened feet and pushed-in ankles. And at the other end your head strains forward to try to bring some balance into this mess. Help is needed!

May we consider once more the Alignment process? It starts with a correction of the feet (not shoes – *feet*). It then works upwards, re-positioning all the parts which would suffer under the additional strains of carrying the unborn baby.

What you do is straightforward. You get your body into a correct alignment as often as possible, whether you are standing, sitting, lying, moving or resting.

Try to *think* re-structured: when you are in a better position, your baby will be in a better position.

And afterwards? If you have kept the Alignment going during your pregnancy, you should be able to move back into a reasonable shape fairly soon. Lying in bed – very shortly after delivery, barring complications – you will do well to get your body in line.

I should like to suggest a series of small movements for you to do in this position when you have a few quiet moments.

Place your hands on your lower abdomen and leave them there. Slowly and gently move your feet so that they are angled outward as far as possible. Hold this position for a moment, slowly bring your feet back to a parallel position, flex your ankles and bring your toes upwards so that they are pointing to the ceiling. Now push your lower back down until it makes contact with the mattress (or floor). Hold this position for about fifteen seconds. Repeat the entire process slowly a few times.

You may also do this in the lying Alignment with your knees flexed up and your feet flat on the mattress/floor. Either way, your feet should be about ten inches apart.

Firstly, this works as a very good starting exercise for strengthening those muscles that have been playing a supporting role for some time.

And, secondly, this will help you to feel your body bringing itself back to normal. You become the owner-occupier once more.

It occurred to me that most of the people looking at my pregnancy pictures will say, 'Oh, she has put more padding in her stomach for the ''wrong'' ones.' Take my word, I am no more padded in 'wrong' than I am in 'right'! The difference lies in the positioning and weight distribution!

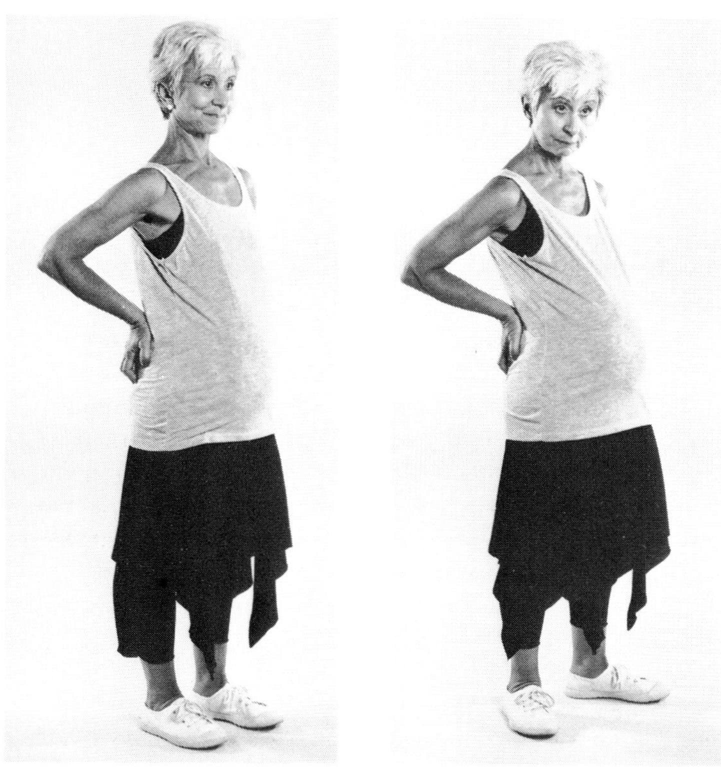

Right **Wrong**

RELAXATION

If the number of different opinions on breathing is impressive, just cast an eye over the subject of relaxation. Since stress became the word-child of big business, relaxation techniques have proliferated, shelf upon shelf, overflowing. If I sound as if I am knocking all this, I am not. We do live in times where stress situations play upon us almost constantly, and where we must find a means of allaying the effects. What I *am* saying, however, is that the means to relaxation have, through the ages, been based on relatively uncomplicated and straightforward principles that have worked quite well. They still do, in most cases, and almost all present-day relaxation techniques are consistent with them.

The important thing is to have a relaxation technique you can use to ease yourself when your emotions or your body cry out. If you already have one that works, fine. However, I should be pleased if you would give mine a try, as it is the natural development of all the work we have done together in this book. It quite simply follows the concept that you are in control through self-knowledge.

My technique is worked through on the same principles as bio-feedback. In the bio-feedback process a machine is used to assist the individual to relax and release tension by pinpointing specific areas of the body. Since you have now worked with your own body in a way that has put you in touch (literally in touch) with each part, you can do the pinpointing on your own. Your owner-occupier familiarity, together with concentration on breathing, is the basis for your relaxation.

The position of the body

You should preferably be lying down. Sitting will do but, particularly after exercise, lying down is best. It's a good idea to align yourself first, then turn your palms to the ceiling and let your ankle joints ease down from their toes-pointed-to-the-ceiling position, so your feet are relaxed. Don't let them flop outwards – this arches the back. If this position – with your legs straight out – is too much of a strain on your back, you may flex your knees up and place your feet parallel to each other and flat on the floor. Close your eyes.

Breathing

You should keep to your own breathing rhythm to start with, using your nostrils to inhale and exhale. Concentrate on the back of the nasal passage as you bring the air in and out. Do this until you can hear your breath moving in and out regularly. Concentrate on the sound. After a few minutes of this, create the word 'release' in your head. Listen more carefully to the exhale and begin to use the word 'release' every time you exhale. Continue in this way for several minutes. Listen (inhale) and 'release' (exhale) – listen (inhale) and 'release' (exhale).

You are breathing regularly and using the word 'release' on the exhale. When you feel eased sufficiently, and want to let go more, start the following touch-memory process.

In your mind remember how the head, neck and all of the vertebrae of the spinal column felt when you touched them. Next create an imaginary line that extends from the crown of the head, down the back of the neck, down the spinal column to the lower back and on to the coccyx. Feel in your mind where each of the parts that line defines is located – back of the head – neck – spine – coccyx.

Holding on to that feel, take a much deeper inhale, filling the lungs but keeping your spine in its flattened position against the floor.

Then on a long *exhale*, using the word 'release', gradually move your mind down that crown-of-head-to-coccyx line, relaxing as you go each part you have located and are holding in your touch-memory: the head – neck – spine – lower back – coccyx. Down, down – resistance out, acceptance in.

Now, slowly, let your mind return to concentrating on the breathing: listen (inhale), 'release' (exhale), listen and 'release'.

The next line will extend from the centre of the forehead, down the nose to the chin, down the centre of the breastbone, the centre of the rib-cage and down to the centre of the abdomen.

In your mind create this line from the centre of the forehead to the centre of the abdomen, locating all of the parts by going back to your touch-memory: nose – chin – breastbone – rib-cage – abdomen.

Listen to your breathing for a moment, then

1. Take a big inhale, and in your mind see the line down the centre.
2. Slowly exhale – and, using the word 'release', mentally move down that centre line easing and relaxing each part along the way.

The method must now be clear, so go back to the breathing – listen, 'release', listen, 'release'.

Next, create lines that extend down both arms, from the shoulders, through the elbows, the wrists and the joints of the fingers, to their very tips.

Keep the pattern of your breathing: listen and 'release', listen and 'release'.

Take a larger inhale, with your lungs lifted and your back flat; then exhale and release (remembering the touch-memory location) from the shoulders all the way down to the tips of the fingers.

You should now be feeling a kind of weightlessness and a oneness with the surface you are lying on.

If you are not, it is of no consequence – just continue to listen, feel, and release.

Next, create a line that runs in front down the centre of the abdomen to the pubis, and another line that runs down the lower back to the coccyx. Think of these two lines as the centres of relaxation for the entire pelvis. Keep to the pattern of breathing.

Then take a bigger inhale, and exhale and release down those lines front and back, extending the touch-memory out to include the hips, the hip joints, the lower abdominal muscles, the cheeks of the buttocks and particularly the lower back.

In releasing the pelvis you may have let your feet angle outwards. If you have, try to direct them in a relaxed way forward, or even slightly in.

Go back to the listen-and-release breathing rhythm again. When you are ready, the next lines will be from the hip joints to the knees, down the shins to the ankle joints.

Mentally see and recall the feel of these parts as you touched them and used them in movements.

Inhale, slowly – see the lines – exhale, slowly – down the lines releasing the parts along the way: hips, knees, ankles.

Now, soothed and relaxed by sound and suggestion, let your mind go to the feet – the first to be aligned, the last to be relaxed.

See them in your mind and remember how they felt.

Take a few breaths. Now draw imaginary lines down the insteps from the centres of the ankle joints to the spaces between the big and second toe. Using an inhale to gather your concentration, send a release on the exhale down the centre line of the instep and across all the joints of the toes. Once more go back to the breathing.

You should now be completely relaxed, but if there is any part still tense or uncomfortable locate it in your touch-memory and apply the exhale/release process once more to this part.

Let yourself float.

It is a very good idea, when you feel you have floated long enough, to 'come out' with the Lying Release and Stretch or perhaps just the Stretch. The chances are you won't fall asleep during the relaxation – you will be too occupied with the process of relaxing – but, if you do, enjoy it!

QUESTIONS OFTEN ASKED

Question: Sometimes I feel that the aligned position makes me look too calculatedly straight. Is it common to feel this?
Answer: Usually people feel this to some degree in the learning stage and when they are getting accustomed to using my Alignment in public. However, the mini-versions are for daily use and once you are familiar with these your sense of self-consciousness should diminish.

Sometimes it is to your advantage to be able to call on looking 'calculatedly straight' in situations where you want to appear very assured and confident, whether in an important business meeting or walking alone on the streets at night.

Question: If I lose weight, how will your Alignment affect the way I look?
Answer: Many people who have had a weight loss still look fat. Losing weight is usually not an answer in itself. A thin body can still have a fat look and requires re-shaping to appear attractively slim. This is one of the things the Norris technique is about. Another is improving muscle tone, which after weight loss is essential.

Question: How does your Alignment technique fit in with visits to chiropractors and osteopaths?
Answer: The Norris Alignment technique teaches you to position your body so that it functions better and acts in preventative and remedial ways for injuries and ills. These are the primary aims and claims of osteopathy and chiropractice,

and undoubtedly on-the-spot relief and corrective positioning are achieved in a high proportion of patients treated. Many of these benefits, however, require a long series of visits and treatments. Good practitioners advise their patients to try to maintain their bodies in correct alignment, but the function of chiropractors and osteopaths is primarily manipulative.

By understanding how to align yourself, you will be able to reinforce the good that has been done and possibly lessen the frequency of return visits. In addition, the value of exercises that practitioners sometimes suggest for supportive muscle development can be heightened by re-structuring your own body first. The entire body, not just associated parts, will be exercised in a position that approximates to the one achieved by manipulation.

Question: How do I know if my feet are aligned when I am wearing shoes?

Answer: Here are some placement pointers that will help you maintain the Alignment in shoes. The first is to be aware of keeping your toes in the straight-ahead/feet-parallel position. This automatically gets a number of things corrected. Another is to check that your ankles are not pushed inwards. You've spent a good deal of time learning how to correct this, but it is a fact that feet stubbornly revert to their old positions more readily when shoes are put on. If you wish, take your hands and make the ankle adjustment, then close your eyes to register the feel. You can do this until the feel becomes so familiar you can make the adjustment without hands – or without looking!

You will probably find that, when lowering or raising your body weight, as in sitting down or getting up, you will be apt to angle out your feet and push in on the ankles (old habits again). Take a look, and make any necessary corrections.

Shoes do tend to inhibit movement of the toes, but it is possible to move those joints and muscles even when confined. Once the toes have been alerted to movement without shoes, you will be able to stretch and place them more correctly in shoes.

Question: How should I position my body when I sleep?
Answer: The best position for sleep is the one you fall asleep in most easily. Unless you have had specific advice to the contrary for medical reasons, you should let preference be the guide. It is, however, a good idea to do your Lying 3-Set before you are in your sleeping position, and certainly the relaxation is an ideal way of ridding yourself of tension preparatory to sleep.

Question: Can I use the Norris technique for on-the-spot relief of specific minor aches and pains?
Answer: I do. Once you realize that the Alignment can take away pain, you can use it whenever you need it. The shoulder rotation permits you to stretch your neck back and relieve tension and discomfort in that area; the hips rotation positions them so that the coccyx can be brought down and the painful pull in the lower back lessened. The very best way to restructure your entire spinal column is to do the Alignment lying on the floor (knees flexed if necessary).

Question: If for some reason I stop practising your Alignment technique on a regular basis, how should I go back to it?
Answer: Although you may have stopped doing your 3-Sets and the other recommended movements on a regular basis, you are probably still using the Alignment on an unconscious basis more than you are aware. The Touch Knowledge introduced you in a palpable way to the logical relationship of your body-parts to one another. This is difficult to dismiss entirely and the body, once initiated into this, will probably retain more active recall than you realize.

To resume a programme, go back once more to read, hear and do the Touch Knowledge. Try it in a warm bath. You do not have to move into a chair. It is all possible sitting in the bath even if a little restricted by the shape. This should put you in touch anew and then the next step is to proceed through Section I. You can set your own pace. Just let your re-reading remind your body and make the necessary commitment to do these things for yourself. Start scheduling your 3-Sets again and proceed with no guilt.

Question: Will I feel any aches and pains when I do your Alignment technique?
Answer: Accurately done, the Norris technique of body alignment should lessen pain and discomfort in the body. However, there is a common tendency to do one thing in the Alignment incorrectly. I shall tell you what it is and how it can be avoided. After the hip rotation and the bringing down of the coccyx, you start the stretch of the torso upwards. In most people the muscles between the upper and lower parts of the body have shortened appreciably and these are the ones that you are stretching at this time. If you attempt to stretch them too much, or too quickly, you will undoubtedly start curving the lower back. If this is happening and you feel pain in that area, STOP. Start the Alignment again and be conscious of not over-stretching to the point of discomfort. In time, and very shortly with continued practice, you will have more body fabric through gradual stretching and even the shoulder rotation will be easier to execute because of this.

One area that may feel as if it has been 'used' – more a feeling of tightness than of anything else – is in the back where the muscles stretch across the shoulder blades. In bringing the shoulders and neck in line these muscles move down into this area to support the back, rather than being strained upwards and tightening the neck. Any discomfort that you feel after the initial re-education of your muscles should last no more than forty-eight hours.

Question: Can I expect 100% improvement when I restructure my body through your technique?

Answer: The extent of the improvement that can be realized is individual. For instance, people with totally flattened arches probably will not be able to lift them, but they can learn to position their feet and ankles so that the condition and its effects are not worsened. An older person who has a 'dowager's hump' may not see a total reduction in its appearance, but continued re-structuring of the body – particularly shoulders and neck – will result in a recognizable improvement in as short a period as three months. This improvement also involves seeing a longer neck! Enlarged joints of the big toes improve as soon as you position your feet so that your weight is not pushed down on them, but in many cases they will not disappear completely.

One thing is certain: by persevering with my technique, most unwanted conditions will be inhibited from worsening, and in many cases there will be improvement to a very considerable degree.

Question: Who can benefit from the Alignment?
Answer: My 'students' come from all walks of life, many of them looking for a remedy to specific problems. Here is a sample of the kind of people who come to me for help.

— A competitive golfer whose lower-back tension was cramping her swing.
— A concert pianist who suffered with arthritic wrists.
— A seeded tennis player who needed help to get her shoulders down and pull in the lower part of her pelvis to add strength and power to her service.
— The owner/manager of a London boutique, who found that after six months of applying Alignment techniques the enlarged joints of her big toes were totally corrected.
— A sculptor who works with a pneumatic drill, who developed severe backache. I showed him how to align himself with his feet straight forward so that he pushes his weight behind his drill from his hips instead of

pushing forward from his lower back.

— A nurse with chronic lower-back pain. I showed her how to lift from her hips when she had to move a patient in bed; and how to stand correctly so that she took the strain off her back and feet.

— The president of an advertising agency with pain in his neck and shoulders from sitting at his desk with his body tensed forward. I showed him how to sit at his desk correctly aligned instead of hunched forward, so that he dominated the stress – and the situation – instead of the stress dominating him.

— Adolescents who have never been taught how to stand up straight properly. Fast growth leaves them uncertain what to do with themselves. They tend to hunch their shoulders. Learning how to align their bodies gives them confidence.

— People who have had illnesses or accidents that have impaired their bodies to the point where exercise is difficult can improve their condition simply by learning how to align themselves.

— People who are bed-ridden and are not using their muscles can be taught to lie in a position that stretches the muscles and exercises them. I give them simple movements they can do lying down which will improve the circulation and keep their muscles flexible.

— Pregnant women suffering from severe backache because no one has told them how to position their feet to alleviate the strain on their lower backs. (As a post-natal exercise, the hip rotation is ideal for helping re-position abdominal muscles.)

— Middle-aged ex-sportsmen who have over-exercised for years and are up to their ears in muscle-bound shoulders. They need help to correct hollow backs and protruding stomachs and to release the tension in their necks and shoulders.

— Middle-aged men and women who have never exercised

but who come to me wanting to get into better shape. They are wary of doing anything too violent in case they injure themselves. Using body alignment techniques, they can start exercising their bodies gradually in order to improve their flexibility and strength.

— Elderly men and women in their seventies and eighties who come to me asking if it is too late to improve their bodies. It is never too late. Correct alignment not only helps to counteract the downward collapse of the body which occurs in later life, it also keeps joints flexible, helping to relieve arthritis, especially in the knees and hip joints.

Question: Is there anyone who should not do your Alignment technique?
Answer: Even if there are physical limitations that are apparent, and my technique cannot be done to its fullest realization, it can be beneficial done on the basis of individual limitation. Even the *attempt* to align the body correctly as this book has taught can work in a therapeutic way.

Question: What should I do to make the Alignment as successful as possible?
Answer: The succinct and straightforward answer is to assume the responsibility for *doing it*. If you actually schedule your 3-Sets regularly, your reminder-bank will grow in proportion. Do them and you will set the pattern to go on doing them. Teach yourself to enjoy the rewards of your own efforts.

A farewell

This book and our work together will provide you with a sensible approach to movement on a life-long daily basis. It also has a carry-it-with-you philosophy that should help to fill your daily needs. I hope it points out that these two do not rely on each other for individual strength but that each can be reinforced by the existence of the other.

To me the really frightened people in this world are the ones who start sentences with 'I always' or 'I never' or, worse still, 'We always'. My message aims to relieve pressures rather than create new ones. There will be days, undoubtedly, when you simply will not want to do the 3-Sets at all. Sometimes you may have an irresistible need to eat an ice-cream cone in a figure S position. Not always – but sometimes. Do enough of the good and you can, with impunity, indulge yourself occasionally with the not-so-good. You've stepped off the path, and hopefully enjoyed it; now all you have to do is step back on.

Life is a balancing act
and you are the juggler

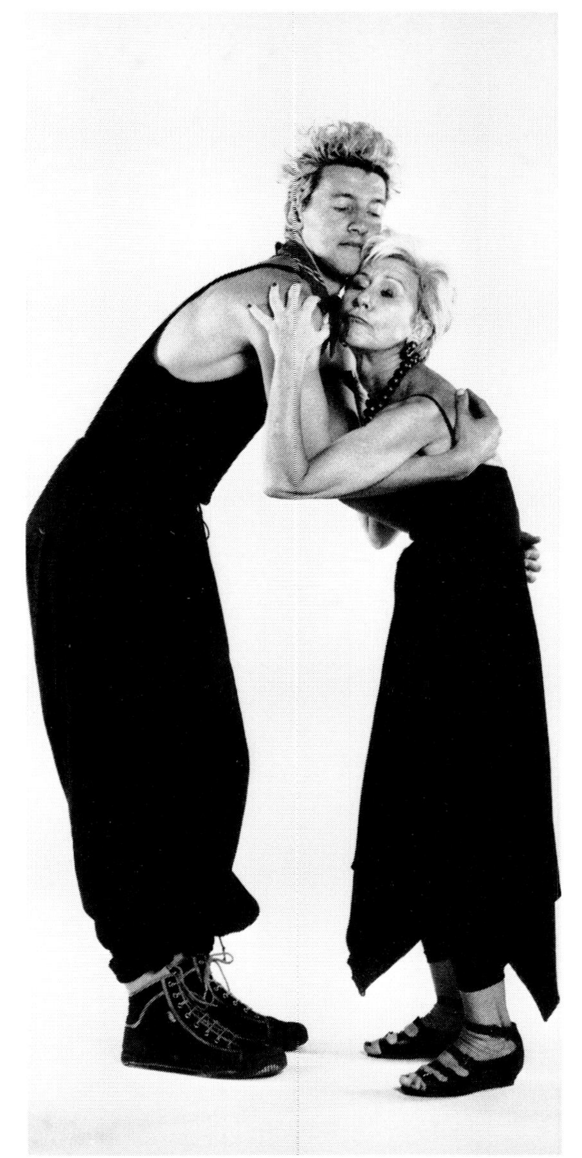

Wrong

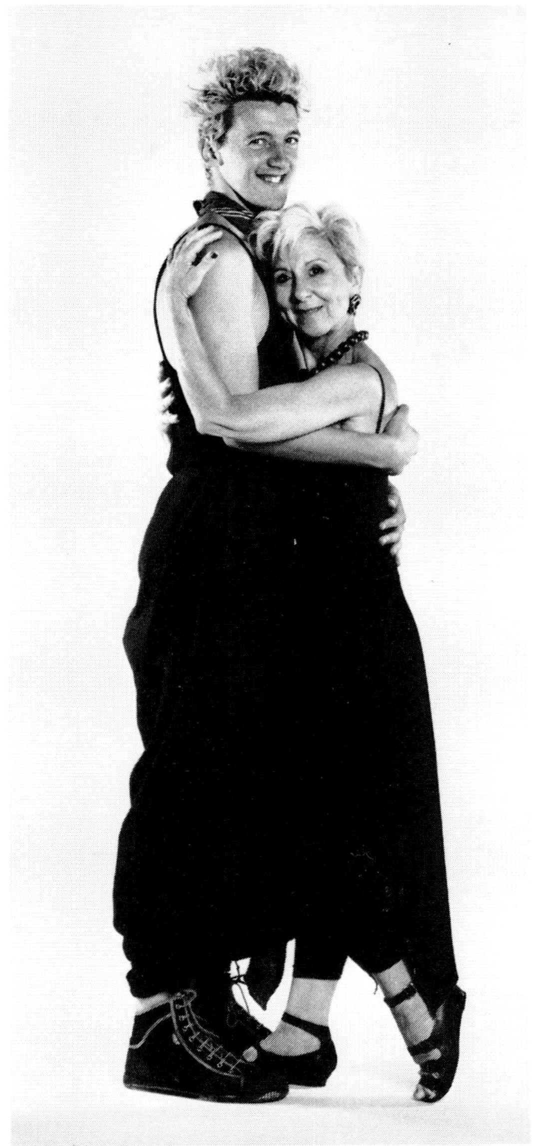

Right

For information regarding the Norris technique of Body Alignment please write to:

14, Broadway
London SW1H 0BH